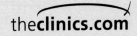

MAGNETIC RESONANCE IMAGING CLINICS

OF NORTH AMERICA

The Lumbar Spine

Guest Editor

DOUGLAS P. BEALL, MD

May 2007 • Volume 15 • Number 2

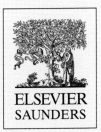

An imprint of Elsevier, Inc
PHILADELPHIA   LONDON   TORONTO   MONTREAL   SYDNEY   TOKYO

W.B. SAUNDERS COMPANY
A Divison of Elsevier Inc.

Elsevier Inc. ● 1600 John F. Kennedy Boulevard ● Suite 1800 ●
Philadelphia, Pennsylvania 19103-2899

http://www.mri.theclinics.com

MRI CLINICS OF NORTH AMERICA Volume 15, Number 2
May 2007 ISSN 1064-9689, ISBN 13: 978-1-4160-4331-7, ISBN 10: 1-4160-4331-4

Editor: Lisa Richman

Reprints: For copies of 100 or more, of articles in this publication, please contact the Commercial Reprints Department, Elsevier Inc., 360 Park Avenue South, New York, New York 10010-1710. Tel. (212) 633-3813, Fax: (212) 462-1935, email: reprints@elsevier.com.

Magnetic Resonance Imaging Clinics of North America (ISSN 1064-9689) is published quarterly by Elsevier Inc., 360 Park Avenue South, New York, NY 10010-1710. Months of issue are February, May, August, and November. Business and Editorial Offices: 1600 John F. Kennedy Blvd., Suite 1800, Philadelphia, PA 19103-2899. Customer Service Office: 6277 Sea Harbor Drive, Orlando, FL 32887-4800. Periodicals postage paid at New York, NY and additional mailing offices. Subscription prices are $226.00 per year (US individuals), $336.00 per year (US institutions), $110.00 per year (US students), $253.00 per year (Canadian individuals), $413.00 per year (Canadian institutions), $149.00 per year (Canadian students), $308.00 per year (international individuals), $413.00 per year (international institutions), and $149.00 per year (international students). International air speed delivery is included in all *Clinics* subscription prices. All prices are subject to change without notice. **POSTMASTER:** Send address changes to *Magnetic Resonance Imaging Clinics*, Elsevier Periodicals Customer Service, 6277 Sea Harbor Drive, Orlando, FL 32887-4800. **Customer Service: 1-800-654-2452 (US). From outside of the US, call 1-407-345-4000.**

Magnetic Resonance Imaging Clinics of North America is covered in the *RSNA Index of Imaging Literature, Index Medicus, MEDLINE,* and *EMBASE/Excerpta Medica.*

Printed in the United States of America.

THE LUMBAR SPINE

GUEST EDITOR

DOUGLAS P. BEALL, MD
Chief of Radiology Services,
Clinical Radiology of Oklahoma;
Director of Musculoskeletal Fellowships;
and Associate Professor of Orthopedic Surgery,
University of Oklahoma, Oklahoma City,
Oklahoma

CONTRIBUTORS

FAISAL ALYAS, FRCR
Fellow, Department of Radiology, Royal National
Orthopaedic Hospital, Stanmore, Middlesex,
London, UK

WALTER S. BARTYNSKI, MD
Associate Professor of Radiology, Department
of Radiology, Division of Neuroradiology,
Presbyterian University Hospital, University
of Pittsburgh Medical Center, Pittsburgh,
Pennsylvania

DOUGLAS P. BEALL, MD
Chief of Radiology Services, Clinical Radiology
of Oklahoma; Director of Musculoskeletal
Fellowships; and Associate Professor of Orthopedic
Surgery, University of Oklahoma, Oklahoma City,
Oklahoma

DAVID CONNELL, FRANZCR
Consultant; and Honorary Clinical Lecturer,
Department of Radiology, Royal National
Orthopaedic Hospital, Stanmore, Middlesex,
London, United Kingdom

RICHARD F. COSTELLO, DO
Chief of Musculoskeletal Radiology, Clinical
Radiology of Oklahoma, Oklahoma City,
Oklahoma

ROSS W. FILICE, MD
Department of Radiology, Johns Hopkins Hospital,
Baltimore, Maryland

JUSTIN Q. LY, MD
Department of Radiology and Nuclear Medicine,
Wilford Hall Medical Center, Lackland Air Force
Base, Texas

DAVID MALFAIR, MD
Clinical Instructor, Division
of Radiology, University of California,
San Francisco, San Francisco,
California

MARK D. MURPHEY, MD
Chief of Musculoskeletal Radiology,
Department of Radiologic Pathology,
Musculoskeletal Division, Armed Forces
Institute of Pathology, Washington,
District of Columbia; Uniformed Services,
University of the Health Sciences, Bethesda,
Maryland

RICK W. OBRAY, MD
Department of Radiology,
Johns Hopkins Hospital, Baltimore,
Maryland

COL PETER S. PALKA, DO
Chief, Neuroradiology; and Chairperson,
Department of Radiology, David Grant Medical
Center, Travis Air Force Base, California

KALLIOPI A. PETROPOULOU, MD
Assistant Professor of Radiology, Department
of Radiology, Division of Neuroradiology,
Presbyterian University Hospital; The Children's
Hospital of Pittsburgh, University of Pittsburgh
Medical Center, Pittsburgh, Pennsylvania

ASIF SAIFUDDIN, FRCR
Consultant; and Honorary Clinical Lecturer,
Department of Radiology, Royal National
Orthopaedic Hospital, Stanmore, Middlesex,
London, United Kingdom

MAJ MICHAEL A. TALL, MD
Chief, Musculoskeletal Radiology; and Program
Director, Radiology Residency, Department
of Radiology, David Grant Medical Center, Travis
Air Force Base, California

ADRIANNE K. THOMPSON, MD
Fellow, MRI, Department of Radiology,
Stanford University School of Medicine, Stanford,
California

TALIA VERTINSKY, MD
Fellow, Body Imaging, Department of Radiology,
Stanford University School of Medicine, Stanford,
California

JORGE A. VIDAL, MD
Junior Scientist in Musculoskeletal Radiology,
Department of Radiologic Pathology,
Musculoskeletal Division, Armed Forces Institute
of Pathology, Washington, District of Columbia

THE LUMBAR SPINE

Volume 15 · Number 2 · May 2007

Contents

Several distinct clinical syndromes can accompany low back pain in patients with
lumbar spine abnormality. Developmental factors and any superimposed degenerative
changes determine the size and configuration of the spinal canal, lateral recess, and
neural foramen, and can affect the nerve roots. Somatic or referred pain may develop
depending on the involved anatomic site and underlying pathology. Many times, but
not always, MR imaging findings correlate with the clinical presentation. Combined
analysis of the imaging and clinical findings may provide a more accurate and concise
approach to the patient with low back pain.

The lumbar spine MR imaging study is one of the most frequently ordered MR imaging
examinations in the United States. Numerous possible causes exist for low back pain,
which contributes to the diagnostic challenge that imagers face in arriving at clinically
relevant diagnoses from the anatomic information provided by MR imaging. In this
article, the authors suggest a systematic approach to MR imaging interpretation. The
evaluation may be altered, based on individual preferences and the specific clinical
scenario. The author also highlights commonly encountered disease processes,
pertinent MR imaging anatomy, and some common diagnostic pitfalls. Normal and
abnormal spine MR images are also shown.

Spine pathology is ubiquitous and is encountered by nearly all medical specialties. The
anatomy of the spine is complex, but the language used to describe pathology may be
even more complex. Many of the common references differ in their nomenclature used
to report intervertebral disk herniation. This article summarizes and relates the standard

recommendations for reporting terminology in regard to herniation of the intervertebral disk. This standard reporting terminology may be used with CT or MR imaging and is useful to report the location and size of the disk herniation. Recommendations are to report abnormalities in zones on axial images and in levels on the sagittal and coronal images. The diagnostician must also be aware of the various pitfalls associated with disk herniation to avoid the scenario of surgical intervention at the incorrect spinal level.

MAJ Michael A. Tall, Adrianne K. Thompson, Talia Vertinsky, and COL Peter S. Palka

Adequate interpretation of a cervical, thoracic, or lumbar spine MR imaging examination includes a careful evaluation of the bone marrow. Detecting an abnormality in bone marrow may cause a diagnostic dilemma because the marrow in the spine can vary in appearance according to the patient's age, and can be affected by infectious, inflammatory, metabolic, and neoplastic processes. Its appearance can be affected as well by underlying degenerative disc disease, trauma, and numerous iatrogenic therapies, including vertebroplasty, radiation therapy, and medications. In addition to conventional MR imaging sequences, newer imaging techniques, such as diffusion weighting and opposedphase sequences, are being studied to help increase the diagnostic accuracy of spine and bone marrow evaluation and to help differentiate benign from malignant and infectious processes.

Faisal Alyas, Asif Saifuddin, and David Connell

The use of MR imaging in assessing lumbar bone marrow first requires an understanding of the bone marrow's normal composition and the various imaging sequences available for use. One of the most useful sequences is the T1-weighted spin-echo sequence. This sequence may be combined with other sequences such as T2-weighted or diffusion-weighted sequences; techniques such as fat suppression, chemical shift imaging, and contrast-enhanced imaging are discussed. The varying features of normal lumbar marrow related to the normal physiologic changes that occur with aging and with changes in hematopoietic demand are important to understand and are described. The appearances of infiltrative marrow disease are explained on the basis of marrow composition and whether disease causes proliferation, replacement, or depletion of normal marrow components.

David Malfair and Douglas P. Beall

Degenerative changes of the spine may involve the disc space, the facet joints, or the supportive and surrounding soft tissues. MR imaging is ideally suited for delineating the presence, extent, and complications of degenerative spinal disease. Other imaging modalities such as radiography, myelography, and CT may provide complimentary information in selected cases. Percutaneous procedures may be used to confirm that a morphologic abnormality is the source of symptoms. Correlation with clinical and electrophysiologic data is also helpful for accurate diagnosis. Combining the information obtained from imaging studies with the patient's clinical presentation is mandatory for determining the appropriate patient management strategy, especially true in patients afflicted with any condition directly attributed to the degenerative processes of the spine.

Jorge A. Vidal and Mark D. Murphey

Primary tumors of the spine are less frequent than metastatic disease, multiple myeloma, and lymphoma. MR imaging is commonly used to evaluate the spine in patients presenting with pain and can further characterize lesions that may be encountered on other imaging studies, such as radiographs, bone scintigraphy, or CT. This article guides radiologists in identifying these lesions and referring physicians to the appropriate patient evaluation. It also offers directions for avoiding all-encompassing broad differential diagnosis lists in situations where the clinical scenario or specific imaging features can significantly limit the diagnostic possibilities.

Rick W. Obray, Ross W. Filice, and Douglas P. Beall

Percutaneous spine intervention, a wide range of invasive spine procedures performed through a puncture hole or through a small incision not requiring soft tissue closure and with few or no skin sutures or staples, is rapidly emerging as an effective alternative to open surgery. This article describes many of the minimally invasive osseous, intervertebral disk, and spinal nerve interventions currently being performed, including both well-established procedures and procedures developed recently. A general introduction to these types of procedures is provided, along with the characteristic pre- and postprocedural MR imaging appearance related to these techniques. The article also discusses reported and theoretical complications that may arise and their respective MR imaging appearances.

GOAL STATEMENT

The goal of *Magnetic Resonance Imaging Clinics of North America* is to keep practicing physicians up to date with current clinical practice by providing timely articles reviewing the state of the art in patient care.

ACCREDITATION

The *Magnetic Resonance Imaging Clinics of North America* is planned and implemented in accordance with the Essential Areas and Policies of the Accreditation Council for Continuing Medical Education (ACCME) through the joint sponsorship of the University of Virginia School of Medicine and Elsevier. The University of Virginia School of Medicine is accredited by the ACCME to provide continuing medical education for physicians.

The University of Virginia School of Medicine designates this educational activity for a maximum of 15 *AMA PRA Category 1 Credits*™. Physicians should only claim credit commensurate with the extent of their participation in the activity.

The American Medical Association has determined that physicians not licensed in the US who participate in this CME activity are eligible for 15 *AMA PRA Category 1 Credits*™.

Credit can be earned by reading the text material, taking the CME examination online at http://www.theclinics.com/home/cme, and completing the evaluation. After taking the test, you will be required to review any and all incorrect answers. Following completion of the test and evaluation, your credit will be awarded and you may print your certificate.

FACULTY DISCLOSURE/CONFLICT OF INTEREST

The University of Virginia School of Medicine, as an ACCME accredited provider, endorses and strives to comply with the Accreditation Council for Continuing Medical Education (ACCME) Standards of Commercial Support, Commonwealth of Virginia statutes, University of Virginia policies and procedures, and associated federal and private regulations and guidelines on the need for disclosure and monitoring of proprietary and financial interests that may affect the scientific integrity and balance of content delivered in continuing medical education activities under our auspices.

The University of Virginia School of Medicine requires that all CME activities accredited through this institution be developed independently and be scientifically rigorous, balanced and objective in the presentation/discussion of its content, theories and practices.

All authors/editors participating in an accredited CME activity are expected to disclose to the readers relevant financial relationships with commercial entities occurring within the past 12 months (such as grants or research support, employee, consultant, stock holder, member of speakers bureau, etc.). The University of Virginia School of Medicine will employ appropriate mechanisms to resolve potential conflicts of interest to maintain the standards of fair and balanced education to the reader. Questions about specific strategies can be directed to the Office of Continuing Medical Education, University of Virginia School of Medicine, Charlottesville, Virginia.

The authors/editors listed below have identified no professional or financial affiliations for themselves or their spouse/partner:
Faisal Alyas, FRCR; Walter S. Bartynski, MD; David Connell, FRANZCR; Richard F. Costello, DO; Ross W. Filice, MD; Justin Q. Ly, MD; David Malfair, MD; Mark D. Murphy, MD; Rick W. Obray, MD; COL Peter S. Palka, DO; Kalliopi A. Petropoulou, MD; Lisa Richman (Acquisitions Editor); Asif Saifuddin, FRCR; Talia Vertinsky, MD; and, Jorge A. Vidal, MD.

The authors/editors listed below identified the following professional or financial affiliations for themselves or their spouse/partner:
Douglas P. Beall, MD (Guest Editor) is an independent contractor, a consultant, on the speaker's bureau, and is on the advisory committee for Medtronic; is an independent contractor, a consultant, and is on the speaker's bureau for Kyphon; is an independent contractor, a consultant, on the speaker's bureau, on the advisory committee, and owns stock in Spineology; and, is a consultant and is on the speaker's bureau for Lilly.
MAJ Michael A. Tall, MD's spouse owns stock in General Electric.
Adrianne K. Thompson owns stock in General Electric.

Disclosure of Discussion of non-FDA approved uses for pharmaceutical products and/or medical devices:
The University of Virginia School of Medicine, as an ACCME provider, requires that all faculty presenters identify and disclose any "off label" uses for pharmaceutical and medical device products. The University of Virginia School of Medicine recommends that each physician fully review all the available data on new products or procedures prior to instituting them with patients.

TO ENROLL

To enroll in the Magnetic Resonance Imaging Clinics of North America Continuing Medical Education program, call customer service at 1-800-654-2452 or visit us online at www.theclinics.com/home/cme. The CME program is available to subscribers for an additional fee of $99.95.

MAGNETIC RESONANCE IMAGING CLINICS

Magn Reson Imaging Clin N Am 15 (2007) xi–xii

Preface

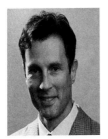

Douglas P. Beall, MD
Guest Editor

Douglas P. Beall, MD
Chief of Radiology Services
Clinical Radiology of Oklahoma
P.O. Box 721688
Oklahoma City, OK 73172-1688, USA

Director of Musculoskeletal Fellowships
Associate Professor of Orthopedic Surgery
University of Oklahoma
610 NW 14th Street
Oklahoma City, OK 73103, USA

E-mail address:
dpb@okss.com

Low back pain is a condition that is near and dear to the vast majority of the adult human population and will be experienced by nearly all individuals during an average lifetime. An issue dedicated to the lumbar spine and the most common manifestation of pathology in this region is intended to not only be professionally informative as to the potential etiologies that can cause low back pain, but is also designed to be of personal interest to many of the readers.

The detection of anatomic derangements in the lumbar spine and the technology that is used to assess the anatomy has improved dramatically. The anatomic assessment is an absolutely vital element in the work-up of patients who have back pain, and it can often lead to a specific anatomic correlate to the patient's clinical symptomatology.

Despite the powerful imaging tools available, the crux of the evaluation is the correlation of the anatomic information with the patient's clinical exam. Unlike the knee, where a large meniscal tear or other anatomic derangement is highly correlative with the presence of clinical symptoms, the lumbar spine may have a host of anatomic abnormalities, and each of these abnormalities may or may not be responsible for the patient's discomfort. The informed comparative assessment is something that is absolutely necessary for each and every patient undergoing an evaluation for low back pain.

The knowledge of common clinical presentations and the anatomic correlate that is most likely to cause these presentations should help in the detection of anatomic pathology when assessing the imaging examinations. A systematic approach to evaluating the lumbar spine should also be applied to produce consistent, accurate, and thorough imaging reports. In addition to visually evaluating the anatomy for the purpose of detecting pathology, the pathology should also be reported in a consistent and conventional manner. The above elements of assessment and reporting have been included in this issue, and manuscripts dealing with some of the most common pathologic processes affecting the lumbar spine, such as degenerative diseases of the spine, intervertebral disk herniations, osseous spinal tumors, and bone marrow

doi:10.1016/j.mric.2007.05.002

disorders have been included. The intent of this issue is to provide the reader with an optimal perspective of the anatomic assessment process, general guidelines of how to report the imaging findings, and informative examples of some of the most common pathologic processes found in the lumbar spine.

A special article included in this issue is the *Magnetic Resonance Imaging of Percutaneous Spine Intervention*. This topic was included because of the dramatic increase in the number and types of percutaneous spine intervention being performed across North America. These minimally invasive procedures are most often performed by physicians, such as radiologists who are familiar with image guided intervention and are comfortable with the visual spacial skill set necessary to navigate the tools within a three-dimensional region while viewing a two-dimensional screen. The knowledge of what these particular procedures accomplish, what a normal post-procedural imaging examination should look like and a familiarity with some of the most common types of complications, will become increasingly necessary as the percutaneous interventional spine procedures continue to proliferate.

Finally, I thank Barton Dudlick, Lisa Richman, Theresa Collier, and the rest of the "Clinics" crew for their tireless work that went into making this issue possible. Their attention to detail, thoughtfulness, and professionalism that went into the review and processing of the manuscripts will undoubtedly be evident to all who have the opportunity to read the manuscripts included within.

ELSEVIER
SAUNDERS

MAGNETIC
RESONANCE
IMAGING CLINICS

Magn Reson Imaging Clin N Am 15 (2007) 137–154

The MR Imaging Features and Clinical Correlates in Low Back Pain–Related Syndromes

Walter S. Bartynski, MD[a],*, Kalliopi A. Petropoulou, MD[a,b]

Low back pain (LBP) and associated clinical syndromes develop as a consequence of four primary factors: pain from the affected spinal element, encroachment of the nerve roots, motion and instability, and irritation related to the expression of inflammatory degenerative disc by-products [1,2].

These elements can be present alone or in combination.

At MR imaging, signal abnormality or a pathologic alteration of anatomy can point to the origin of axial LBP. In addition, spinal canal shape changes can help predict potentially compressed or

[a] Department of Radiology, Division of Neuroradiology, Presbyterian University Hospital, University of Pittsburgh Medical Center, 200 Lothrop Street, D132, Pittsburgh, PA 15213, USA
[b] The Children's Hospital of Pittsburgh, University of Pittsburgh Medical Center, 200 Lothrop Street, D132, Pittsburgh, PA 15213, USA
* Corresponding author.
E-mail address: bartynskiws@upmc.edu (W.S. Bartynski).

symptomatic nerve roots that contribute to the patient's overall pain pattern. This article reviews the anatomic features that either relate to axial pain or relate to the acquired secondary symptoms of axial pain, such as radiculopathy.

Spine innervation and low back pain

Spine pain is related to the pattern of spinal innervation. Ventral spinal elements (disc/annulus, anterior longitudinal ligament [ALL], posterior longitudinal ligament [PLL], vertebral body, epidural plexus, and dura) are innervated separately from posterior spinal elements (facet joints, spinous process, ligamentum flavum, and posterior muscles), and the local pain from these two groups is often distinct [3–10]. Recently, more convincing evidence of direct annular innervation by nociceptive fibers has become available, which further establishes the intervertebral disc as a direct potential contributor to the development of LBP [11,12].

Disc, vertebral body, posterior longitudinal ligament, epidural plexus, and dura

In the ventral spine, pain sensation is believed to be transmitted centrally by way of two major pathways with separate but overlapping fiber networks: somatic pain fibers and sympathetic pain fibers (Fig. 1A, B) [4–10].

Somatic pain fibers are found along the dura, epidural venous plexus, PLL, and posterior annular margin. These fibers enter the sinuvertebral nerve, project to the dorsal root ganglion, and then extend to the cord (see Fig. 1A) [5–10].

Sympathetic pain fibers are considered the primary nociceptors of the anterior vertebral structures (ALL, anterior and lateral annulus).These fibers receive branches through the gray ramus communicans (or anterior spinal ramus) and project to the paraspinal sympathetic ganglion (see Fig. 1B). In the more posterior ventral structures (PLL and posterior annulus), sympathetic pain fiber innervation is present with branches entering the sinuvertebral nerve and projecting to the paraspinal sympathetic

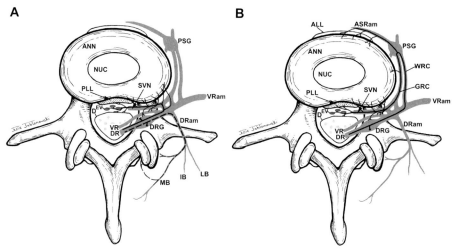

Fig. 1. Spine Innervation. (*A*) Somatic nociceptive innervation and the dorsal ramus. Somatic nociceptive innervation is received from the posterior longitudinal ligament, posterior annulus, epidural venous plexus, and ventral dura. Fibers course through the sinuvertebral nerve (*solid lines*) to the dorsal root ganglion and finally to the cord and brain. Posteriorly, the dorsal ramus is comprised of three branches: median, intermediate, and lateral. The median branch of the dorsal ramus receives nociceptive supply from spinal elements including the facet joint, lamina, spinous process, and posterior ligaments; it also supplies the multifidus muscle (*dashed lines*). The intermediate and lateral branches supply lateral muscles and receive supply from the skin. (*B*) Sympathetic nociceptive innervation. The anterior and posterior longitudinal ligaments, annulus, and vertebral body are supplied by sympathetic nociceptive fibers (*solid lines*). These fibers course to the paraspinal sympathetic ganglion from either the anterior spinal sympathetic ramus (anteriorly) or the sinuvertebral nerve and gray ramus communicans (posteriorly). After reaching the paraspinal sympathetic ganglion, fibers pass to the dorsal root ganglion, through the white ramus communicans, and eventually to the cord and brain. The gray ramus is variable and the white ramus is inconstant below L2. ALL, anterior longitudinal ligament; ANN, annulus; ASRam, anterior paraspinal sympathetic ramus; D, dura; DR, dorsal root; DRam, dorsal ramus; DRG, dorsal root ganglion; EV, epidural veins; GRC, gray ramus communicans; IB, intermediate branch; LB, lateral branch; MB, median branch; NUC, nucleus pulposus; PLL, posterior longitudinal ligament; PSG, paraspinal sympathetic ganglion; SVN, sinuvertebral nerve; VR, ventral root; VRam, ventral ramus; WRC, white ramus communicans.

ganglia through the gray ramus communicans. The sympathetic fibers exit the paraspinal sympathetic ganglion, course through the white ramus communicans, enter the dorsal root ganglion, and ultimately project to the cord. Central sympathetic pain fiber transmission is somewhat variable and may extend along the paraspinal sympathetic ganglia before entering the canal, because presence of the gray ramus communicans can vary, and the white ramus communicans are inconstant below L2 [10].

Facet, ligamentum flavum, lamina, spinous process, and interspinous ligament

Posterior or dorsal innervation is supplied by the dorsal ramus with the presence of three main branches—the median branch, intermediate branch and lateral branch—which are often distinguished by their muscular supply (see Fig. 1A) [7,8,10]. The median branch is the primary supply of the facet joint, interspinous ligament, spinous process, and multifidus muscle, with sparse contribution to the ligamentum flavum. The facet is innervated by contributions from both adjacent median branches. Intermediate branches from adjacent levels form a network and innervate the longissmus thoracis muscle; lateral branches receive sensory input from the lumbar and upper-lateral gluteal skin and supply the iliocostalis lumborum muscle [7].

Nerve root

Innervation of the nerve root and dorsal ganglion region is taken primarily from local somatic and sympathetic fiber supply (see Fig. 1A, B) [10]. Both somatic and sympathetic pain responses can be noted with dermatomal distribution as well as nondermatomal or referred pain patterns previously referred to as the "zones of head" (Fig. 2).

With isolated compression, the nerve root generally responds with loss of function with resultant weakness, loss of deep tendon reflexes in the muscle groups supplied, and paresthesia, tingling, and burning in the associated dermatome. When the root is irritated by compression or chemicals, it becomes edematous, and local stimulation (eg, direct postoperative testing, laminectomy under local anesthetic, nerve block procedures) results in provocation of the radicular pain response [13–15].

Spinal canal shape changes and associated clinical syndromes

As lumbar structures are affected by arthritis/disease, changes occur in the shape of the disc/endplate, facet joint, capsule ligaments, or ligamentum flavum. These shape changes lead to

alteration in the size or shape of the spinal canal and neural foramen with resultant neural compression. Nerve root, cauda equina, or spinal cord encroachment can lead to a group of distinct clinical syndromes. These features can be further aggravated by subluxation or shape changes induced by weight bearing or upright posture.

Clinical presentations

Radiculopathy

Isolated nerve root compression or irritation leads to a complex series of changes that result in radiating leg pain (see Fig. 2). This pain can have a dermatomal distribution extending along the path of the dermatome, consistent with a nerve root's skin sensory supply [16,17]. Alternatively, referred radiating pain may develop from adjacent structures, which

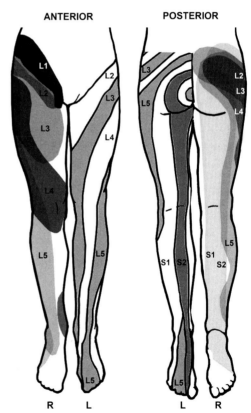

Fig. 2. Patterns of radiating leg pain (radiculopathy). Radiating leg pain can appear dermatomally (left leg, front and back) or may be referred by other spine nociceptors. The referred pain is complex and likely centrally processed with a variable nondermatomal representation in the leg, which is inconstant from side to side and inconstant between people (right leg, front and back). These have been previously called the "radiating zones of head". (*Data from* Refs. [10,16–18].)

follow the entire somatome (with more complete dermatomal, myotomal, and sclerotomal contributions) and presents with more nonspecific distribution [10,16,18]. Termed the "radiating zone of head," the somatomal patterns of radiating pain are less specific, are likely processed centrally in the cord or brain, fail to follow dermatomal innervation, and may parallel the vascular supply to the leg. Overlap of these patterns can occur and variations in accepted patterns of dermatomal innervation exist, which make prediction of the involved root problematic [10,14,16–18].

Innervation of the lower extremity is related to the individual nerve roots and the distribution provided by the lumbar plexus. While individual dermatomal regions exist, variation in presentation makes exact targeting difficult. In addition to somatic and sympathetic pattern effects, segmentation anomaly/variation occurs (approximately 8% in the lumbo-sacral region), which leads to further radiculopathy variation [19]. In general, upper lumbar radicular symptoms presenting above the knee (ie, L3, L4) can be separated from lower root symptoms presenting with pain below the knee (ie, L5, S1), but exact root targeting can be difficult. In addition, multiple roots may contribute to radicular pain, which further confuses the presentation.

A series of companion physical findings develop in response to direct nerve root compression: power loss in muscle groups of the affected nerve, loss in deep tendon reflexes of the affected segment, and paresthesia in the dermatome (Table 1) [17]. Pain is commonly accentuated by leg and foot extension (straight leg raising sign), which is either related to a stretch of the irritated sciatic nerve or worsening impingement of the root in the corners of the spinal canal [17,20]. Intrinsic sciatic nerve irritation may be present with pain in the gluteal and hip region and can be accentuated by direct palpation.

It is well known that root compression can be present without symptoms [21]. Pain is often absent, and in spite of anatomic distortion, there is no objective loss of power, abnormal deep tendon reflexes, or paresthesia. Therefore, the anatomic distortion is an indicator of potential root dysfunction and radiculopathy, but is not an absolute.

In addition, chemical irritation (presumably from degenerative disc byproducts) may occur with radiating leg pain in the absence of anatomic distortion [22–25]. This irritation can be reversed by applying local anesthetic, which is what typically occurs after nerve block or steroid injection application.

Neurogenic claudication

In patients who have peripheral vascular disease, vascular claudication can develop because of poor arterial circulation; leg and calf pain develops after walking short distances (1–2 blocks) and is relieved by rest. Patients who have chronic lumbar stenosis and cauda equina compression frequently present with a nearly identical clinical pattern that has been called "neurogenic claudication" [26–28]. These patients also complain of leg and calf pain or cramping after walking short distances. There is one major difference between these patients and those who have vascular claudication: the patients who have neurogenic claudication need to sit, squat, or bend over for pain relief, which allows spinal canal flexion/expansion and reduced cauda equina compression. Walking downhill can provoke symptoms whereas walking uphill tends to be easier. Additional complaints in patients who have cauda equina compression include gait difficulty, variable and nonspecific paresthesia, and occasional bladder dysfunction.

Conus compression and acute cauda equina syndrome

Conus compression typically leads to expression of upper motor neuron signs and weakness, in addition to any element contributing to local back pain [29]. The hallmark includes hyperreflexia accompanied by a positive Babinski sign (ie, the classic "upgoing great toe" when the plantar reflex is stimulated). In acute conus compression, flaccid rectal tone and urinary retention typically accompany paresis. In chronic compression, hyperreflexia and peripheral atrophy are present.

Table 1: Typical motor and sensory radicular patterns

Root	Typical motor loss	Typical sensory location	Reflex arc
L2	Hip flexion	High anterior thigh	None
L3	Knee extension	Mid-anterior thigh	Adductor
L4	Foot inversion	Anterior thigh to knee	Knee jerk
L5	Toe dorsiflexion	Posterior thigh, calf, ankle, dorsum foot	None
S1	Foot plantar flexion, eversion	Posterior thigh, calf, lateral foot	Ankle jerk

In acute cauda equina syndrome, the compression typically leads to asymmetric paresis and sensory loss with areflexia [29]. Sphincter dysfunction may also occur.

Anatomic patterns of compression

The development of root compression depends upon the initial shape and size of the spinal canal, lateral recess, or neural foramen coupled with the development of superimposed degenerative changes or pathology. In some patients, the size of the spinal canal is intrinsically small (congenital stenosis), and a lesser degree of degenerative change may produce symptomatology in these patients.

Lateral recess

At the pedicle level, the spinal canal can have either an open triangular shape or trefoil configuration (Fig. 3). If the shape is initially trefoil, the nerve root is located in the "niche" or "lateral recess" of the canal [30,31]. If the shape is initially triangular, facet/ligament hypertrophy and any associated disc bulge/end plate spur can lead to an acquired niche or lateral recess shape [30,31]. Further narrowing of the congenital or acquired lateral recess niche will result in nerve root impingement and compressive radiculopathy [30–33]. A bony lateral recess height of less than 3 mm is considered suggestive of lateral recess stenosis and a recess less than 2 mm is considered diagnostic [30].

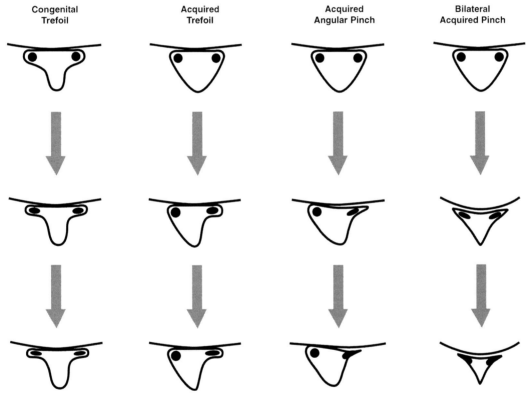

Congenital Trefoil   Acquired Trefoil   Acquired Angular Pinch   Bilateral Acquired Pinch

Fig. 3. Development of the lateral recess, central spinal stenosis, and lateral recess stenosis. Congenital trefoil canal: the lateral recess region becomes progressively narrowed due to either facet or endplate disc margin degenerative changes. Acquired trefoil canal: early facet degenerative changes and hypertrophy in a triangular canal develops a trefoil shape with the root positioned in a lateral recess niche. Progressive disc margin, endplate, or further facet degenerative changes lead to compression of the trapped root. Acquired angular pinch (of the lateral recess): simultaneous and equal facet, endplate, and disc margin degenerative changes lead to acute angle formation in the corner of the canal and lateral recess region. The root becomes progressively compressed in the lateral recess and may be medially deflected. Bilateral acquired angular pinch (of the lateral recess): bilateral facet, disc margin, and endplate degenerative changes can narrow the central spinal canal and the lateral recess region. This can produce both central spinal stenosis with cauda equina compression and individual nerve root compression within the abnormal lateral recess. (*Adapted from* Bartynski WS, Lin L. Lumbar root compression in the lateral recess: MR imaging, conventional myelography and CT myelography comparison with surgical confirmation. AJNR Am J Neuroradiol 2003;24:349, © American Society of Neuroradiology; with permission.)

The central spinal canal

If a patient's spinal canal was originally open and triangular, degenerative changes of the facet and intervertebral disc can narrow the canal in a uniform fashion at the disc/facet level. Uniform spinal canal narrowing will result in the small triangular shape associated with central spinal stenosis (see Fig. 3). The degree of canal narrowing can be mild, moderate, or severe, and with significant compression of the cauda equina, neurogenic claudication can develop. Antero-posterior spinal canal diameter less than 12 mm in size is considered strongly suggestive of stenosis [26–28,32,34].

Progressive degenerative changes in the presence of lateral recess stenosis (congenital or acquired) can also lead to a small triangular shape with both central cauda equina compression and isolated root compression in the niche (see Fig. 3) [31,32]. These changes could result in neurogenic claudication, radiculopathy, or both.

The neural foramen and far lateral region

The size and shape of the neural foramen can be altered with the development of disc and facet degeneration. Disc height loss, bulge, protrusion, or end plate spur combined with facet hypertrophy and ligament thickening can lead to focal root/ganglion compression or circumferential foraminal narrowing/compression and radiculopathy (Fig. 4).

Foraminal distortion can also develop with subluxation, especially when combined with degenerative disc changes and/or facet changes. With subluxation, the pedicle changes position and overlays the exposed (uncovered) disc and annular margin (Fig. 4C). Loss of disc height accompanied by disc degeneration leads to earlier root and ganglion compression because of this unique anatomic arrangement. The addition of focal disc protrusion or presence of an extruded fragment can affect the root earlier because of the pre-established small foraminal size. Compressive radiculopathy results in typical radiating leg pain.

Intervertebral disc

The shape and location of disc degenerative changes can play a role in the radicular symptoms that develop. Although nomenclature will be reviewed in other articles in this issue, several points are pertinent to a patient's clinical presentation.

Disc disease can affect groups of nerve roots an individual nerve root, depending on the size and location of the protrusion/extrusion/sequestration (Fig. 5). The line of demarcation is the medial

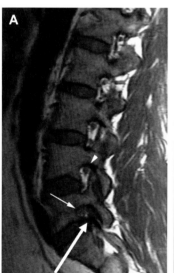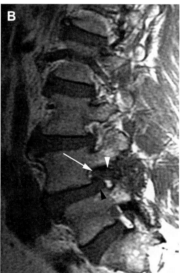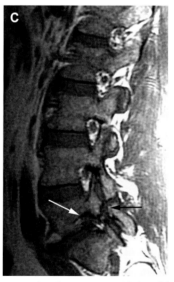

Fig. 4. Root compression in the neural foramen. (*A*) Significant foraminal narrowing is present at L5-S1 with early root distortion (*small white arrow*) and compression caused by degenerative disc changes with loss of disc height and mild bulge of the disc margin (*large white arrow*). This is contrasted with the normal foraminal appearance at L4-5 where the root is visible just under the L4 pedicle with fat and vessels in the lower aspect of foramen (*arrowhead*). (*B*) With degenerative spondylolithesis and facet hypertrophy, early compression of the L4 root is present in the L4-5 foramen (*white arrow*). Disc height loss, slight protrusion of the disc margin (*black arrowhead*), and anterolisthesis cause the swollen root to be compressed between the pedicle and the exposed disc. Further compression is contributed by the L4-5 superior facet capsule redundancy (*white arrowhead*). (*C*) With spondylolysis (*black arrow*) and disc degeneration, the nerve root becomes trapped between the forwardly positioned pedicle and the uncovered disc margin (*white arrow*) caused by the loss of disc height.

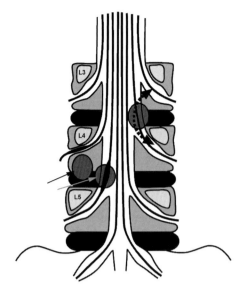

Fig. 5. Spinal canal and foramen compression: disc migration. A disc protrusion, extrusion, or sequestration isolated to the neural foramen/far lateral region affects the nerve root/ganglion as it courses beneath the pedicle and beyond (ie, L4 as it passes beneath the L4 pedicle [*black arrow*]). Paracentral disc protrusion, extrusion, or sequestration that remains within the spinal canal (generally medial to the pedicle) affects the nerve root as it traverses the disc margin (ie, L5 as it passes by the L4-5 disc margin [*gray arrow*]). If the protrusion is both paracentral and foraminal it can affect the traversing root and the root in the foramen, which gives a mixed radicular response. A paracentral extrusion that migrates can also affect two roots by projecting inferiorly to the lateral recess or superiorly to the pedicle as demonstrated at L3-L4 (*curved broken arrows*).

pedicle border (MPB). If the protrusion is lateral to the MPB and isolated to the neural foramen or far lateral region, the root and ganglion exiting under the pedicle will be effected (ie, the L4 root exiting under the L4 pedicle at the L4-5 level). Focal paracentral protrusion lying medial to the MPB typically interacts with the traversing nerve root still in the spinal canal before exiting the neural foramen below, which causes a separate pattern of radiculopathy (ie, the L5 root at the L4-5 level as it begins to course toward the L5 pedicle). A disc that subtends both the lateral spinal canal and neural foramen can develop radicular symptoms from both roots with a portion of the symptoms contributed from each.

A large paracentral extrusion/sequestration can also migrate superiorly or inferiorly and affect the root in the canal (as it passes the disc margin) and the root in the neural foramen (above) or lateral recess (below). If a protrusion, extrusion, or sequestration is large and the spinal canal is small

(congenital or acquired), compression of the cauda equina can occur and neurogenic claudication can develop.

Spinal alignment and subluxation

Altered spinal alignment can affect both the neural foramen and spinal canal in a variety of ways that lead to cauda equina or isolated root compression. Subluxation is often associated with degenerative disc disease, and discogenic pain can develop in addition to pain from motion.

The effects of spondylolisthesis (anterolisthesis) depend upon the presence or absence of spondylolysis. Spondylolisthesis without spondylolysis is typically caused by facet degeneration/remodeling with central spinal canal, lateral recess, and foraminal narrowing caused by anterior shift of the lamina/facets along with disc height loss. Spondylolisthesis with spondylolysis typically develops root compression because of disc uncovering, associated disc height loss, and resultant foraminal narrowing with the root compressed between the pedicle and uncovered disc margin.

Considering the above-mentioned factors, subluxation from degenerative spondylolisthesis results in canal narrowing and stenosis with foreword migration of posterior elements (Fig. 6A). Subluxation from spondylolysis results in an enlarged canal due to the posterior elements remaining behind (Fig. 6C). This anatomic arrangement can best be visualized in the sagittal plane [35]. Other causes of subluxation (trauma) could render a mixture of these features.

Imaging protocols

Classic and established MR imaging protocols usually assess the lumbar spine anatomy or signal changes that reflect lumbar pathology. Both T1-weighted and T2-weighted sequences in the sagittal and axial planes are generally routine. Fat saturation in the sagittal T2 commonly is used to assess bone lesions or edema surrounding the posterior elements. Post contrast T1-weighted images with fat saturation in at least one plane contribute to better assessing entities such as discitis, osteomyelitis, or postoperative spine. Sequences such as gradient echo or diffusion-weighted imaging may be part of a more tailored protocol to detect certain pathologies.

Sagittal sequences are more informative if all foramina are fully covered. The axial sequences can be acquired along the plane of each disc or following one best angle. Both techniques have their advantages. Axial images display the disc ideally on one slice. However, one must cover from pedicle to pedicle at each level to allow consistent evaluation of the lateral recess. Discontinuous scanning,

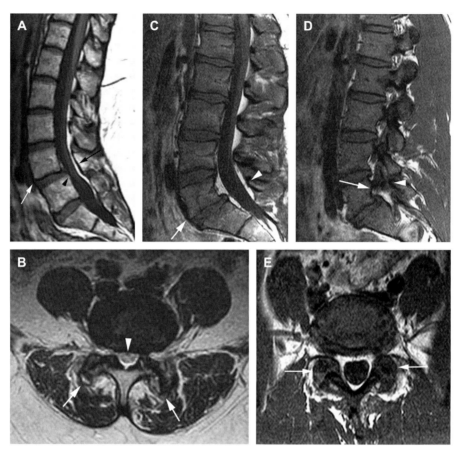

Fig. 6. Subluxation: spondylolisthesis and spondylolysis. (*A*) Sagittal midline T1-weighted MR image of a patient who has degenerative spondylolisthesis at L4-5. The vertebral body and posterior elements move anteriorly (*white and black arrows*) leading to progressive narrowing of the spinal canal with resultant stenosis (*arrowhead*). (*B*) Axial T2-weighted MR image of this patient demonstrates severe facet degenerative changes and remodeling (*arrows*) with severe spinal stenosis caused by the anterior position of the posterior elements with small anterior–posterior canal diameter (*arrowhead*) along with facet joint degenerative change and hypertrophy. (*C*) Sagittal midline T1-weighted MR image of a patient who has spondylolisthesis with spondylolysis and LBP demonstrates anteriolisthesis of the L5 vertebral body (*arrow*). The posterior elements of L5 remain behind, which leads to spinal canal widening (*arrowhead*). (*D*) Sagittal off lateral T1-weighted MR image of this patient with L5-S1 spondylolysis with spondylolisthesis. The pars defect (*arrowhead*) is best noted in the sagittal plane with the L5 nerve root seen approaching the L5-S1 foramen narrowed by loss of disc height, low position of the pedicle, and the bulging uncovered disc margin (*arrow*). (*E*) In the axial plane, the spondylolysis can mimic a facet joint (*arrows*) if one is not careful to recognize the absence of a complete posterior ring in the stack of axial images at the involved interspace.

performed when angling the plane along the intervertebral discs, can also result in missed disc fragments if not combined with a continuous axial slice sequence.

Clinical conditions: imaging and clinical pattern correlates

Disc degeneration and discogenic pain

It has been debated whether the intervertebral disc is truly an independent source of LBP. Laminectomy performed under local anesthetic or upon postoperative anatomic testing demonstrated that the annulus can be painful [13–15]. Now innervation of the peripheral annulus is established and recent publications support the presence of nociceptive pain fibers in the outer portion of the annulus [5,7]. Pain fiber innervation likely reaches the peripheral 1/3 of the normal annulus, and it seems to extend to the inner annulus and perhaps even into the nucleus as degenerative changes develop [7,11,12]. Therefore, discogenic pain is becoming more fundamentally grounded as a process that has a firm pathoanatomic correlate.

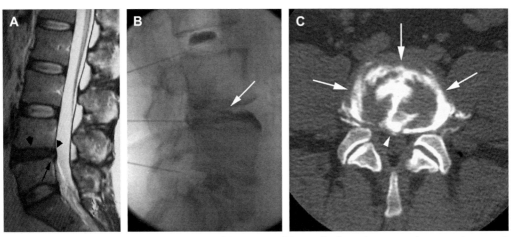

Fig. 7. Disc degeneration and discogenic pain. This 49-year-old man had persistent LBP for several years when the pain was recently exacerbated by an injury. (A) Sagittal T2-weighted MR image demonstrates significant degenerative disc changes at L4-5 with decreased disc height and bulge of the posterior disc margin (*arrowheads*). Reduced disc signal is consistent with disc desiccation and altered proteoglycan composition with a small focal hyperintense zone present along the posterior disc margin, which suggests an annular tear (*black arrow*). (B) Contrast injection at L4-5 during discogram provoked the man's typical/familiar lumbar pain. Discogram fluoroscopic image demonstrates significant intradiscal derrangement with annular tears and annular/nuclear fragmentation (*arrow*). (C) Postdiscogram CT demonstrates complex and severe peripheral annular tears (*arrows*) and a radial tear with contrast extravasation from annular leakage (*arrowhead*). The radial tear projects to the canal surface of the disc margin and is likely consistent with the hyperintense zone noted on the sagittal MR image (*arrowhead*). Intradiscal lidocaine administration substantially relieved the patient's provoked pain.

Imaging features associated with degenerative disc disease have been well established. Signal changes reflecting altered water content and altered proteoglycans are best noted on the sagittal T2-weighted imaging with reduced disc signal, reduced disc height, and bulge of the disc peripheral margin (Fig. 7A). Changes in marrow signal may develop because of a reaction to the adjacent disc degeneration, which suggests marrow edema, fat replacement, or fibrosis. Disc protrusion, extrusion, or sequestration can occur with more advanced degenerative changes.

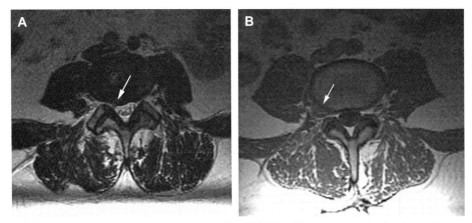

Fig. 8. Focal disc protrusion and nerve root compression. (A) Disc with canal compression (traversing root). This patient has right L4 radiculopathy. An axial T2-weighted image demonstrates right-sided paracentral disc protrusion at L3-4 with isolated compression of the L4 nerve root in the lateral canal as it traverses the disc margin (*arrow*). (B) Disc with foramen compression (foraminal root). Patient with right-sided L4 radiculopathy. An axial T1-weighted image demonstrates a right foraminal and far lateral disc protrusion with isolated compression of the L4 root in the lateral foramen (*arrow*). Patient obtained complete relief from his radiculopathy from L4 nerve root block and steroid administration.

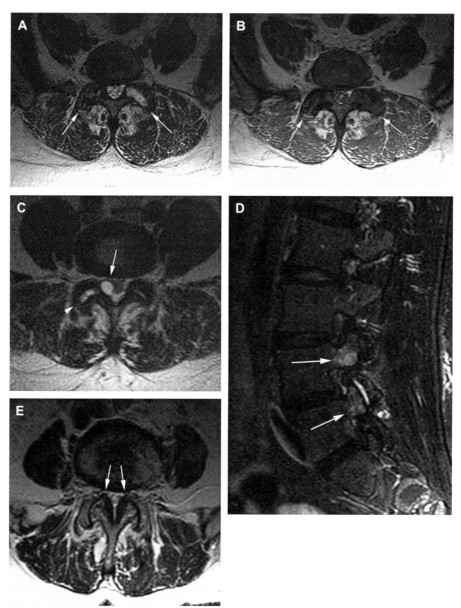

Fig. 9. Facet arthropathy. (*A, B*) Facet pain and degenerative facet disease. Axial T2-weighted and T1-weighted images in these focally painful facets were more typical of advanced disease (*arrows*) and were bilaterally responsive to local anesthetic and steroid administration. The painful facet joint can have features of more recent inflammation but is typically benign in appearance, with hypertrophy and spur formation predominating. Facet fluid can be present but is extensive only in the face of subluxation or synovial cyst formation. (*C*) Facet pain and synovial cyst. Fluid accumulation in the joint can occur (*arrowhead*) with facet degeneration. Synovial outpouching can occur either within the spinal canal or externally with progressive joint expansion. When a synovial cyst forms in the spinal canal, compression of the thecal sac or adjacent nerve root can occur, which contributes to radiculopathy (*arrow*). (*D*) Facet pain with accompanying marrow edema. This patient presented with a painful L4-5 facet joint, and marrow edema can be seen in the adjacent pedicles (*arrows*). In general, the edema is restricted to the bone, but it can incite a reaction in the adjacent soft tissues with some capsular or paraspinal inflammation, which can be difficult to separate from infection. (*E*) Lateral recess stenosis with radiculopathy. Axial T2-weighted MR image demonstrates facet hypertrophy and disc bulge at L4-5 with acquired lateral recess stenosis bilaterally with L5 root impingement (*arrows*): worse on the left. The patient had only right-sided L5 radiculopathy that completely resolved with transforaminal L5 nerve root block and steroid injection.

Patients who have degenerative disc disease typically describe deep or dull aching LBP; sharp, stabbing, knife like pain; or both, which are common symptoms of L4-5 and L5-S1 (90%). Both types of pain may be provoked with certain movements or provocative discography [36–39]. Motion or position change is commonly associated with pain provocation and may play a role in the presentation. At discography, disc degeneration demonstrates features of annular or nuclear fragmentation; annular, radial, or peripheral circumferential tears; and potential leakage of the intradiscal contents into the foramen or epidural space (Fig. 7B, C). Identification of the hyperintense zone in the posterior peripheral annular margin of the intervertebral disc is a sign that is most likely related to LBP (see Fig. 7A) [40,41]. Basic imaging features may reflect a painful disc but are less specific.

While disc bulging simply may reflect degenerative changes and loss of disc height, it can also be associated with radicular symptoms. If the lateral recess is narrow, for example, the root passing the disc can become entrapped and radicular symptoms develop.

Focal disc protrusion, extrusion, and sequestration

Typically superimposed on the MR imaging features of disc degeneration, focal disc protrusion, extrusion, or sequestration demonstrate the eccentric shape of the disc margin or clear evidence of disc material projecting from the disc into the canal. With disc protrusion, extrusion, or sequestration, pain from root compression is typically superimposed on longstanding or acute pain from the disc [17].

Two different clinical nerve root presentations may develop, depending on the location of the protrusion, extrusion, or sequestration relative to the traversing or exiting nerve roots (Fig. 8A, B). The critical factor is whether the disc protrusion affects the root in the spinal canal as it passes by the disc margin (ie, L5 at the L4-5 disc space), or whether it encroaches in the neural foramen and affects the root as it lies under the pedicle (ie, L4 at the L4-5 disc space). These impingement scenarios also may overlap and combine to render blended root presentations. A large protrusion or extrusion may cause stenosis and neurogenic claudication.

Facet joint arthropathy, synovial cyst, and degenerative spondylolisthesis

Symptomatic facets typically demonstrate features of long-standing facet degeneration (Fig. 9A–C). Facet hypertrophy and spur formation usually are superimposed on changes in the size of the spinal canal or neural foramina and commonly occur in conjunction with features of degenerative disc disease [42]. Facet joint effusion may be present, and chronic facet effusions may give rise to facet joint cysts that can extend into the spinal canal or posteriorly outside of the spinal canal [43]. Thickening or hypertrophy of the ligamentum flavum almost always develops in conjunction with degenerative hypertrophy of the facet joints. Occasionally, marrow edema is apparent, and the edema may track into the adjacent pedicle [42].

Degenerative spondylolisthesis usually is associated with a degenerative disc disease (see Fig. 6A, B). The facet joint is typically abnormal in shape (with significant hypertrophy and degeneration) and shifted anteriorly in position. Focal disc protrusion also may be present (seen in 4%–20% of patients), and the combination of spondylolisthesis and disc protrusion may be associated with symptomas of radiculopathy [44].

Clinically, the abnormal symptomatic facet joint may result in LBP. This pain is typically elicited by direct palpation, may change with flexion and extension, and responds well to local anesthetic and steroid administration [42]. This pain pattern also is noted at the painful sacroiliac joint. Spinal canal distortion, which commonly develops as a result of hypertrophic facet degeneration (and is often associated with disc degenerative changes), leads to central canal narrowing and stenosis with the potential for producing neurogenic claudication. Isolated nerve root entrapment in the lateral recess of the canal or in the neural foramen also may occur as a result of hypertrophic degenerative changes of the facet joints and can result in symptoms of radiculopathy.

Central spinal stenosis

The imaging findings of central spinal stenosis include a small intrinsic canal size (either resulting from congenital or acquired stenosis) and other degenerative features that contribute to acquired spinal stenosis; these features include degenerative disc disease, degenerative facet disease, and spondylolisthesis (Fig. 10). With mild stenosis, only a minor canal shape change may be apparent. With severe stenosis, cerebrospinal fluid (CSF) may no longer be visible at the level of the encroachment. In addition, nerve and vessel redundancy may be apparent above and below the level of the stenosis, along with prominent epidural fat and a prominent epidural venous plexus. Stenosis also may increase with extension and weight bearing, which can be seen with myelography or weight bearing MR imaging (Fig. 10A, B) [45–47].

Although spinal canal size may not be a reliable predictor of symptoms, patients who have chronic stenosis usually develop neurogenic claudication

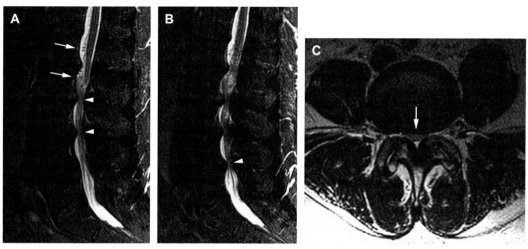

Fig. 10. Spinal stenosis. (*A*) Sagittal MR image in a patient with neurogenic claudication. Significant spinal canal narrowing with root compression is apparent at L2-3 and L3-4 (*arrowheads*); nerve root redundancy also is noted above the stenotic levels (*arrows*). (*B*) After simulated weight bearing with a compression device, an additional level of severe stenosis is noted at L4-5 (*arrowhead*) with worsening stenosis at L2-3 and L3-4. (*C*) Axial MR image at L4-5 demonstrates severe spinal stenosis due to congenitally short pedicles and asymmetric disc bulge with central compacting of the nerve roots and complete elimination of CSF in the stenotic region (*arrow*).

and radiculopathy superimposed on LBP. In acute stenosis, which can occur with a large extruded disc, patients may develop cauda equina syndrome.

Spondylolysis and spondylolisthesis

Spondylolysis is typically bilateral (85%–90%) and usually presents at L5 (80%). Spondylolysis, also known as a pars defect, can produce LBP related either to the pars abnormality or the resultant subluxation and degenerative disc changes (see Fig. 6) [48]. Imaging demonstrates anterolisthesis but with a widened spinal canal. Associated degenerative changes can result in disc height loss with further encroachment of the neural foramen (see Fig. 6D). Degenerative changes at the defect (Gill's nodule) and within the facet joints may develop,

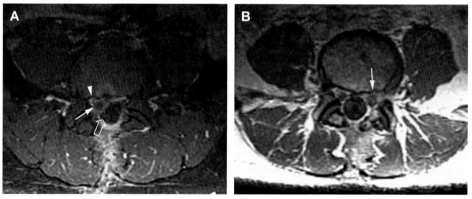

Fig. 11. Postoperative pain. (*A*) Postoperative recurrent disc. Recurrent disc protrusion typically occurs because of fragmentation of residual annulus with extrusion through the operative site. Compression of the adjacent nerve root typically elicits radiculopathy. On the postcontrast T1-weighted image, a recurrent fragment is noted just below the L4-5 disc space near the disc margin as a focal nonenhancing fragment surrounded by enhancing an epidural scar (*arrow*). The L5 nerve root (*arrowhead*) and thecal sac (*open arrow*) are compressed, and an L5 nerve root block rendered complete pain relief. (*B*) Postoperative epidural scar. Epidural enhancement adjacent to the annular margin and surrounding the traversing nerve root is frequently observed after discectomy (*arrows*). This patient, who had midline laminectomy/discectomy at L4-5, had some residual left-sided radicular pain considered referable to the L5 nerve root. The patient improved completely with transforaminal L5 nerve root block and steroid administration.

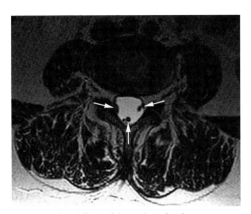

Fig. 12. Arachnoiditis. This patient had numerous episodes of sepsis and hip joint infections requiring multiple open debridement operations. She now has nonspecific LBP with radiating leg pain. Nerve root clumping and dural adherence is noted consistent with arachnoiditis (*arrows*).

from a preoperative disc protrusion with a combination of LBP and radiculopathy (Fig. 11A). If pain from recurrent disc herniation persists, another discectomy may be required.

Postoperative pain associated with fibrosis is typically a mixture of residual LBP and radiating leg discomfort, which are symptoms typical of radiculopathy. Targeted nerve root block and steroid administration are frequently helpful in finding the origin of the pain, and they are often used to control both the local back pain and the radiating leg pain components (Fig. 11B).

After fusion, the clinical features of persistent or recurrent pain can be more complicated. Pain may persist at the operative level but is more often associated with accelerated degenerative changes above or below the fusion with disc degeneration, disc protrusion, or the development of canal stenosis.

which leads to focal spinal canal narrowing and radiculopathy.

Post laminectomy and discectomy pain

Postoperative infection rarely occurs after discectomy, but recurrent disc herniation and postoperative scarring are common [49]. Pain from recurrent disc herniation is similar to pain

Arachnoiditis

Arachnoiditis was common in the oil-based myelography era, but it is encountered only occasionally today. MR imaging demonstrates intrathecal nerve root and arachnoid inflammation with root-to-root adhesions, root-to-dural adhesions, and intrathecal cyst formations (Fig. 12) [49]. Arachnoiditis may be characterized by nonspecific LBP,

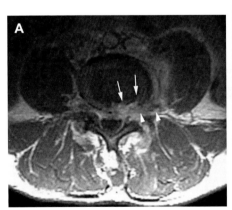

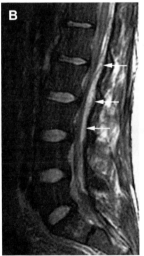

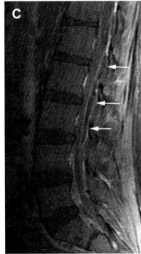

Fig. 13. Infection. (A) Discitis with foramen encroachment and radiculopathy. Typically presenting with LBP without associated findings, this patient also developed left-sided radiculopathy with severe radiating leg pain. Discitis is clearly present with disc and vertebral marrow signal abnormality (*arrows*). Paraspinal inflammation is also present, projecting into the neural foramen (*arrowheads*), and is responsible for the patient's left radiculopathic pain component. The organism in this patient was methcillin-resistant *Staphylococcus aureus*. (B, C) Epidural abscess. This patient developed severe LBP, right leg pain, and methcillin-resistant *S aureus* bacteremia from intravenous drug abuse. Sagittal T2-weighted and post contrast T1-weighted MR imaging on admission demonstrated an extensive epidural collection in the posterior spinal canal (*arrows*) with obvious thecal sac and cauda equina compression that ultimately required surgical drainage.

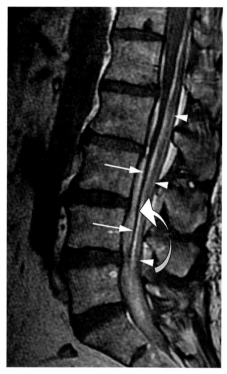

Fig. 14. Spontaneous epidural hemorrhage. Extradural blood is dissecting through the ventral and dorsal epidural space (ventral *arrows* and dorsal *arrowheads*) in this patient, who presented with severe knife like LBP, mixed lower extremity weakness, and paresthesias with early bowel and bladder dysfunction. The thecal sac is compressed in a circumferential fashion and appears as only a thin low-signal ribbon in the center of the spinal canal (*widened curved arrow*).

spastic paraparesis, nonspecific radiating leg discomfort, and dysesthesias.

Vertebral infection

The clinical patterns associated with vertebral infection are often nonspecific. In adults, discitis typically begins with focal vertebral osteomyelitis and extends into the avascular disc space. LBP is the typical presenting complaint, but radiculopathy can develop if foraminal extension is present (Fig. 13A). Fever is often absent, and the white blood cell count may be variable. Constitutional symptoms may be present, and bacteremia may be detectable if blood cultures are obtained. Elevation of the erythrocyte sedimentation rate is considered the most reliable laboratory abnormality [50].

With significant epidural phlegmon or abscess formation, foraminal or canal compromise can develop and result in severe radiculopathy, neurogenic claudication, or acute cauda equina syndrome. Paraspinal or psoas abscess formation can lead to irritation of the lumbar plexus. This irritation can produce features of psoas irritation with leg guarding and muscular spasm.

An epidural abscess can develop in an equally insidious fashion, which predominately creates symptoms of nonspecific LBP until objective neurologic signs of root or cauda equina compression are apparent (Fig. 13B, C) [51,52].

Spontaneous epidural hemorrhage

Spontaneous epidural hemorrhage is uncommon and usually found in the cervicothoracic region [53]. Patients with lumbar epidural hemorrhage typically present with severe, lancinating, knifelike LBP and radicular symptoms and an imaging

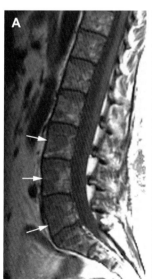
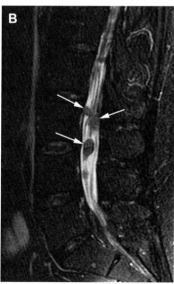

Fig. 15. Spine tumors. (*A*) Bone lesions with bone pain. This 51-year-old patient had acute lymphoblastic leukemia and developed severe LBP with some leg pain. MR imaging shows multiple bone lesions consistent with bony leukemic infiltration (*arrows*). (*B*) Drop mets with root pain. This patient had lung carcinoma and developed persistent bilateral leg pain. MR imaging showed multiple large intrathecal nerve root drop metastases (*arrows*).

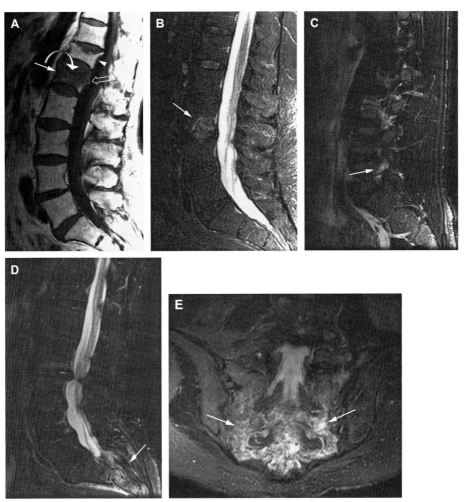

Fig. 16. Vertebral injury. Although vertebral compression fracture is a common cause of pain caused by vertebral injury, acute Schmorl's node formation can also occur. Additionally, injury may be present in more subtle areas that require the observer to inspect the edges of anatomy covered on the imaging study, such as pedicle injury and sacral insufficiency fracture. (*A*) Acute osteoporotic vertebral compression fracture. Evidence of an acute L1 vertebral body compression is present with collapse of the superior endplate (*curved arrow*) and some buckling of the posterior vertebral margin (*open arrow*). Marrow edema is noted with uniform decreased signal on T1-weighted images; an increased signal was also present on T2-weighted images (*straight white arrow*). In contrast, an older vertebral compression fracture at T12 is noted with abnormal shape but normal marrow appearance (*arrowhead*). (*B*) Acute LBP and Schmorl's node. Focal collapse of the inferior endplate of L3 is apparent in this patient who has acute LBP (*arrow*). Adjacent marrow edema is present and is similar to a vertebral compression fracture, but it is restricted to the focally deficient and injured inferior endplate. (*C*) Pedicle stress injury with edema. Focal LBP was present in this competitive gymnast. The pedicle stress injury is observed best on the post fat saturation T2-weighted image, commonly obtained in the sagittal plane, but must be carefully looked for at the edges of the imaging study (*arrow*). (*D, E*) Sacral insufficiency fracture. A sacral insufficiency fracture can be a subtle but important cause of LBP, especially in elderly patients (*arrows*), and is often noted on the off center sagittal T2-weighted image at the most inferior aspect of the spine. Diffuse marrow edema was present in this patient, but it can be restricted to the sacral alar region and difficult to appreciate in the midline.

appearance suggesting recent or variably aged blood byproducts dissecting through the epidural space (Fig. 14). The patient may have a known coagulopathy related to anticoagulant therapy, chemotherapy, hepatic dysfunction, or transplantation; or a laboratory assessment may reveal an unexpected alteration in the patient's prothrombin time, partial thromboplastin time, or platelet level.

Spine tumors

The most common tumor of the spine is metastatic disease and, like infection, it can present with both central axial back pain and radiating leg pain, depending on what structures are being affected. Tumor extension to the osseous cortical surface or associated vertebral collapse likely will be associated with central back pain because of innervation of the vertebral body periosteum. Extension beyond the vertebral body with adjacent root encroachment can also lead to a typical radiculopathic presentation (Fig. 15A).

Tumors of the conus or cauda equina can occur with variable clinical presentations. A combination of leg pain, back pain, and paresthesia can occur due to root infiltration by tumor, root encroachment, vertebral compressive remodeling, or intratumoral hemorrhage. Foraminal tumors such as a neurinoma or a meningioma frequently present with radicular symptoms and radicular pain caused by root encroachment.

Patients with carcinomatous meningitis or drop metastases can develop back pain and either subtle or overt radicular symptoms (Fig. 15B). Cerebral spinal fluid cytology and MR imaging are complimentary in establishing the diagnosis [54,55].

Vertebral injury

Lumbar osteoporotic vertebral compression fractures are common and typically present with focal nonspecific LBP that may be quite focal to percussion (Fig. 16A) [56–58]. Wedge deformity, vertebral flattening, and marrow edema are the hallmark MR imaging findings. Spinal stenosis, lateral recess stenosis, or neural foraminal encroachment can occur with vertebral collapse, leading to neurogenic claudicaiton or radiculopathy. Progressive degenerative changes of the adjacent disc and facets can develop, which makes detection of the primary cause of patient pain confusing. Acute Schmorl's node formation can also present with nonspecific LBP. The focal endplate fracture, the hallmark of the Schmorl's node, can have associated focal marrow edema (Fig. 16B) [59].

Stress injury of the pedicle (Fig. 16C) or sacral insufficiency fracture (Fig. 16D, E) can be subtle on MR imaging [60]. Marrow edema may be present and either suggest or support the diagnosis. Bone scan can be helpful in controversial cases or when further confirmation is necessary.

Summary

Clinical pain patterns that develop in the lumbar spine depend upon the primary source of the pain. Anatomic derangements can provide clues to potential areas of pain generation and associated deformities of the spinal canal, lateral recesses, and neural foramina; these symptoms may present with radiculopathy or neurogenic claudication.

Attention to the imaging patterns and potential areas of root or cauda equina compression can help support the clinical impression and target the appropriate treatment more accurately.

Acknowledgment

The authors thank Eric Jablinowski for his support with artwork and contribution to image preparation.

References

[1] Cavanaugh JM. Neural mechanisms of lumbar pain. Spine 1995;20:1804–9.
[2] Siddall PJ, Cousins MJ. Spinal pain mechanisms. Spine 1997;22:98–104.
[3] Sherman MS. The nerves of bone. J Bone Joint Surg 1963;45:522–8.
[4] Jackson HC, Winkelmann RK, Bickel WH. Nerve endings in the human lumbar spinal column and related structures. J Bone Joint Surg Am 1966;48:1272–81.
[5] Bogduk N, Tynan W, Wilson AS. The nerve supply to the human lumbar intervertebral discs. J Anat 1981;132(Pt 1):39–56.
[6] Bogduk N, Wilson AS, Tynan W. The human lumbar dorsal rami. J Anat 1982;134:383–97.
[7] Bogduk N. The innervation of the lumbar spine. Spine 1983;8:286–93.
[8] Groen GJ, Baljet B, Drukker J. The innervation of the spinal dura mater: anatomy and clinical implications. Acta Neurochir (Wien) 1988;92:39–46.
[9] Groen GJ, Baljet B, Drukker J. Nerves and nerve plexuses of the human vertebral column. Am J Anat 1990;188:282–96.
[10] Jinkins RJ. The pathoanatomic basis of somatic and autonomic syndromes originating in the lumbosacral spine. Neuroimaging Clin N Am 1993;3:443–63.
[11] Freemont AJ, Peacock TE, Goupille P, et al. Nerve ingrowth into diseased intervertebral disc in chronic back pain. Lancet 1997;350:178–81.
[12] Ozawa T, Ohtori S, Inoue G, et al. The degenerated lumbar intervertebral disc is innervated primarily by peptide-containing sensory nerve fibers in humans. Spine 2006;31:2418–22.
[13] Falconer MA, McGeorge M, Begg C. Observations on the cause and mechanism of symptom-production in sciatica and low back pain. J Neurol Neurosurg Psychiatr 1948;11:13–26.
[14] Smyth MB, Wright V. Sciatica and the intervertebral disk. An experimental study. Clin Orthop Relat Res 1977;129:9–21.
[15] Kuslich SD, Ulstrom CL, Michael CJ. The tissue origin of low back pain and sciatica: a report of pain response to tissue stimulation during operations on the lumbar spine using local anesthesia. Orthop Clin North Am 1991;22:181–7.

[16] Chusid JG. Correlative neuroanatomy and functional neurology. Los Altos (CA): Lang Medical Publications; 1982.

[17] Standaert CJ, Herring SA, Sinclair JD. The patient history and physical examination: cervical thoracic and lumbar. In: Herkowitz HN, Garfin SR, Eismont FJ, et al, editors. Rothman-Simeone: the spine. 5th edition. Philadelphia: Sauders Elseivier; 2006. p. 171–86.

[18] Mooney V, Robertson J. The facet syndrome. Clin Orthop Relat Res 1976;115:149–56.

[19] Korber J, Bloch B. The "normal" lumbar spine. Med J Aust 1984;140:70–2.

[20] Smith SA, Massie JB, Chesnut R, et al. Straight leg raising. Anatomic effects on the spinal nerve root without and with fusion. Spine 1993;18:992–9.

[21] Jensen MC, Brant-Zawadzki MN, Obuchowski N, et al. Magnetic resonance imaging of the lumbar spine in people without back pain. N Engl J Med 1994;331:69–73.

[22] Olmarker K, Rydevik B, Nordborg C. Autologous nucleus pulposus induces neurophysiologic and histologic changes in porcine cauda equina nerve roots. Spine 1993;18:1425–32.

[23] Gronblad M, Virri J, Tolonen J, et al. A controlled immunohistochemical study of inflammatory cells in disc herniation tissue. Spine 1994;19:2744–51.

[24] Saal JS. The role of inflammation in lumbar pain. Spine 1995;20:1821–7.

[25] Olmarker K, Blomquist J, Stromberg J, et al. Inflammatogenic properties of nucleus pulposus. Spine 1995;20:665–9.

[26] Verbiest H. A radicular syndrome from developmental narrowing of the lumbar vertebral canal. J Bone Joint Surg Br 1954;36:230–7.

[27] Ehni G. Significance of the small lumbar spinal canal: cauda equina compression syndromes due to spondylosis. Part 1: introduction. J Neurosurg 1969;31:490–94.

[28] Amundsen T, Weber H, Lilleas F, et al. Lumbar spinal stenosis. Clinical and radiologic features. Spine 1995;20:1178–86.

[29] Fehlings MG, Dandie GDC, Ng WP. Clinical syndromes of spinal cord disease. In: Barjer HH, Loftus CM, editors. Textbook of neurological surgery. Philadelphia: Lippincott Williams & Wilkins; 2003. p. 1577–83.

[30] Mikhael MA, Ciric I, Tarkington JA, et al. Neuroradiological evaluation of lateral recess syndrome. Neuroradiology 1981;140:97–107.

[31] Bartynski WS, Lin L. Lumbar root compression in the lateral recess: MR imaging, conventional myelography and CT myelography comparison with surgical confirmation. AJNR Am J Neuroradiol 2003;24:348–60.

[32] Epstein JA, Epstein BS, Rosenthal AD, et al. Sciatica caused by nerve root entrapment in the lateral recess: the superior facet syndrome. J Neurosurg 1972;36:584–9.

[33] Ciric I, Mikhael MA, Tarkington JA, et al. The lateral recess syndrome. A variant of Spinal stenosis. J Neurosurg 1980;53:433–43.

[34] Epstein JA, Epstein NE. Lumbar spondylosis and spinal stenosis. In: Wilkins RH, Rengachary SS, editors. Neurosurgery. 2nd edition. New York: McGraw-Hill; 1996. p. 3831–40.

[35] Ulmer JL, Elster AD, Mathews VP, et al. Distinction between degenerative and isthmic spondylolisthesis on sagittal MR images: importance of increased anteroposterior diameter on the spinal canal (wide canal sign). AJR Am J Roentgenol 1994;163:411–6.

[36] Walsh TR, Weinstein JN, Spratt KF, et al. Lumbar discography in normal subjects. A controlled, prospective study. J Bone Joint Surg Am 1990; 72:1081–8.

[37] Milette PC, Raymond J, Fontaine S. Comparison of high-resolution computed tomography with discography in the evaluation of lumbar disc herniations. Spine 1990;15:525–33.

[38] Moneta GB, Videman T, Kaivanto K, et al. Reported pain during lumbar discography as a function of anular ruptures and disc degeneration. A re-analysis of 833 discograms. Spine 1994;19: 1968–74.

[39] Derby R, Howard M, Grant JM, et al. The ability of pressure-controlled discography to predict surgical and nonsurgical outcomes. Spine 1999; 24:364–71.

[40] Aprill C, Bogduk N. High-intensity zone: a diagnostic sign of painful lumbar disc on magnetic resonance imaging. Br J Radiol 1992;65(773): 361–9.

[41] Schellhas KP, Pollei SR, Gundry CR, et al. Lumbar disc high-intensity zone. Correlation of magnetic resonance imaging and discography. Spine 1996;21:79–86.

[42] Czervionke LF, Fenton DS. Facet joint injections and medial branch block. In: Fenton DS, Czervionke LF, editors. Image-guided spine intervention. Philadelphia: Saunders; 2003. p. 9–49.

[43] Metellus P, Fuentes S, Adetchessi T, et al. Retrospective study of 77 patients harbouring lumbar synovial cysts: functional and neurological outcome. Acta Neurochir (Wein) 2006;148:47–54.

[44] Epstein NE. Far lateral and foraminal lumbar disc herniations. In: Barjer HH, Loftus CM, editors. Textbook of neurological surgery. Philadelphia: Lippincott Williams & Wilkins; 2003. p. 1661–7.

[45] Nowicki BH, Yu S, Reinartz J, et al. Effect of axial loading on neural foramina and nerve roots in the lumbar spine. Radiology 1990;176:433–7.

[46] Inufusa A, An HS, Lim TH, et al. Anatomic changes of the spinal canal and intervertebral foramen associated with flexion-extension movement. Spine 1996;21:2421–10.

[47] Willen J, Danielson B. The diagnostic effect from axial loading of the lumbar spine during computed tomography and magnetic resonance imaging in patients with degenerative disorders. Spine 2001;26:2607–14.

[48] Logroscino G, Mazza O, Aulisa AG, et al. Spondylolysis and spondylolisthesis in the pediatric

and adolescent population. Childs Nerv Syst 2001;17:644–55.

[49] Ross JS. MR imaging in the postoperative lumbar spine. Magn Reson Imaging Clin N Am 1999; 7(3):513–24.

[50] Cahill DW, Abshire BB. Pyogenic vertebral osteomyelitis. In: Barjer HH, Loftus CM, editors. Textbook of neurological surgery. Philadelphia: Lippincott Williams & Wilkins; 2003. p. 3239–47.

[51] Nussbaum ES, Rigamonti D, Standiford H, et al. Spinal epidural abscess: a report of 40 cases and review. Surg Neurol 1992;38:225–31.

[52] Chang FC, Lirng JF, Chen SS, et al. Contrast enhancement patterns of acute spinal epidural hematomas: a report of two cases. AJNR Am J Neuroradiol 2003;24:366–9.

[53] Groen RJM. Non-operative treatment of spontaneous spinal epidural hematomas: a review of the literature and a comparison with operative cases. Acta Neurochir (Wein) 2004;146:103–10.

[54] Larson DA, Rubenstein JL, McDermott MW. Treatment of metastatic cancer. In: DeVita VT, Hellman S, Rosenberg SA, editors. Cancer, principles & practice of oncology. 7th edition. Philadelphia: Lippincott Williams & Wilkins; 2005. p. 2323–36.

[55] Chamberlain MC. Neoplastic meningitis: a guide to diagnosis and treatment. Curr Opin Neurol 2000;13:641–8.

[56] Jensen ME, Evans AJ, Mathis JM, et al. Percutaneous polymethylmethacrylate vertebroplasty in the treatment of osteoporotic vertebral body compression fractures: technical aspects. AJNR Am J Neuroradiol 1997;18:1897–904.

[57] Barr JD, Barr MS, Lemley TJ, et al. Percutaneous vertebroplasty for pain relief and spinal stabilization. Spine 2000;25:932–28.

[58] Evans AJ, Jensen ME, Kip KE, et al. Vertebral compression fractures: pain reduction and improvement in functional mobility after percutaneous polymethylmethacrylate vertebroplasty-retrospective report of 245 cases. Radiology 2003;226:366–72.

[59] Takahashi K, Miyazaki T, Ohnari T, et al. Schmorl's nodes and low back pain. Eur Spine J 1995;4:56–9.

[60] Dasgupta B, Shah N, Brown H, et al. Sacral insufficiency fractures: an unsuspected cause of low back pain. Br J Rheumatol 1998;37:789–93.

ELSEVIER
SAUNDERS

MAGNETIC
RESONANCE
IMAGING CLINICS

Magn Reson Imaging Clin N Am 15 (2007) 155–166

Systematic Approach to Interpretation of the Lumbar Spine MR Imaging Examination

Justin Q. Ly, MD

The lumbar spine MR imaging study is one of the most frequently ordered MR imaging examinations in the United States, a reflection not only of a high prevalence of low back pain but of the recent advancements in MR imaging technology that allow accurate detection and depiction of spine pathology. Numerous possible causes exist for low back pain (lumbago), which contributes to the diagnostic challenge that imagers face in arriving at clinically relevant diagnoses from the anatomic information provided by MR imaging. Determining cause is further complicated by the fact that low back pain is often multifactorial and that anatomic abnormalities may not necessarily translate into clinical symptoms. As a result, imaging physicians accept that in most cases, only a probable cause for the back pain can be suggested, and it remains critically important for the referring clinician to correlate abnormal MR imaging findings with the patient's clinical findings. To maximize the usefulness of the imaging evaluation to the patient and to the referring clinician, a systematic approach should be used during every MR imaging interpretation of the lumbar spine. The following suggested

approach is only one of many possible approaches the imager can invoke, and the evaluation may be altered, based on individual preferences and the specific clinical scenario. Although this article is not intended to be a comprehensive written or pictorial review of lumbar spine pathology, the authors also highlight commonly encountered disease processes, pertinent MR imaging anatomy, and some common diagnostic pitfalls. Normal and abnormal spine MR images are also shown, but a detailed discussion of all aspects of lumbar spine MR imaging, including technical considerations, pulse sequences, postoperative spine appearance, and nomenclature of intervertebral disc disease, is beyond the scope of this particular article.

Discussion

A systematic approach can encourage a thorough evaluation of the spine and can help avoid overlooking portions of the anatomic evaluation when scrutinizing an MR imaging evaluation of the lumbar spine. The following sequential evaluation of the anatomic elements of the lumbar spine may

Department of Radiology and Nuclear Medicine, Wilford Hall Medical Center, 2200 Bergquist Drive, Suite 1, Lackland Air Force Base, TX 78236-5300, USA
E-mail address: jly15544@hotmail.com

1064-9689/07/$ – see front matter © 2007 Elsevier Inc. All rights reserved.
mri.theclinics.com

doi:10.1016/j.mric.2007.04.002

be used to ensure a complete and consistent evaluation.

General overview

An initial assessment of the lumbar spine should begin with an overall appearance appraisal. What is the overall or general condition of the spine, as demonstrated on the sagittal images (and coronal images if obtained)? Quickly, one should be able to identify any gross evidence of recent trauma or metastatic disease, or evidence of a diffuse, marrow-involving process; whether the presence of a tumor or infection should be considered; or if the case is simply one characterized by the various types of degenerative change (the most common scenario encountered). As part of the initial overall appearance assessment, a gross idea of the severity of the disease process should be formulated. The sagittal T2-weighted or short T1 inversion recovery (STIR) images can be a good place to start. (Fig. 1 shows normal sagittal spine anatomy).

Assessment of vertebral alignment/ligaments

Immediately after the overall appearance appraisal, one may assess the vertebral alignment. Do all of the vertebral bodies maintain a normal relationship with the adjacent vertebral body and are they appropriately aligned (ie, are the contiguous anterior, posterior, and lateral cortices aligned as well as would be expected)? In the setting of recent trauma, a finding of malalignment requires exclusion of an associated fracture. In the absence of acute trauma, the most common cause of abnormal vertebral body alignment or vertebral body subluxation is degenerative spondylolisthesis.

Spondylolisthesis of one vertebral body in relationship to another may be in any direction but the most common direction is anterior spondylolisthesis, where one vertebral body is anteriorly displaced in relation to another. Defects in the pars interarticularis portion of the vertebrae (thought to be related to either a congenital deficiency or chronic repetitive microtrauma) should also be considered, especially when an anterior spondylolisthesis is detected (Fig. 2A). Defects of the pars interarticularis are most common at the L4 and L5 levels and may be associated with the presence of sclerosis or callus formation adjacent to the regions of the defects.

Detection of pars defects on MR imaging examinations may not be easy and it may be difficult to differentiate between prominently narrowed pars interarticularis structures that contribute to degenerative spondylolisthesis and a frankly fractured pars interarticularis that subsequently produces spondylolisthesis caused by spondylolysis (a complete bony defect of the pars interarticularis). Pars

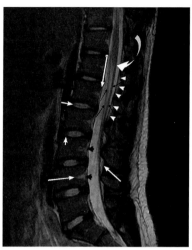

Fig. 1. Midsagittal T2-weighted MR image with fat saturation of the lumbar spine in a young adult male patient. The tip of the conus medullaris is located at the mid-T12 level (*curved white arrow*), with demonstration of normal appearance of cauda equina nerve roots (*black arrows*). Thin, dark posterior longitudinal ligament (*long white arrow directed caudad*) is in direct continuity to the anterior aspect of the thecjal sac. Posterior aspect of the thecal sac is thin and dark (*series of arrowheads*), with epidural fat located directly posterior (*oblique white arrow*). Note the sharp zone of transition (*short white arrow directed cephalad*) between the well-hydrated nucleus pulposus and the dark annulus fibrosis; this crisp demarcation is preserved in young patients. Linear, low-signal intranuclear cleft is an early sign of degeneration (*short white arrow directed posterior*). More subtle fibrous intranuclear cleft is also seen at the disc level immediately below. Elongated, triangular high T2 signal at the posterior aspect of the L4 vertebral body represents fat around the basivertebral plexus (*long arrow pointing posteriorly*), with Batson's plexus representing the high T2 signal directly posterior/adjacent to the posterior vertebral body cortex (*black arrowheads*).

interarticularis thinning or destruction has been classified by at least two different MR imaging classification systems. The region of the pars is best seen with either sagittal T1-weighted, or two- or three-dimensional gradient echo, images and the morphology of the pars is usually determined on one of these imaging series.

One classification, or grading, system grades the degree of pars involvement by whether or not the bone marrow signal is continuous through the pars (grade 1), whether the pars has bony sclerosis (grade 2), or whether it is indeterminate (grade 3) [1]. This same classification system distinguishes between a single-sided cortical discontinuity (grade 4a) and a cortical discontinuity that involves both the anterior and posterior portions of the pars

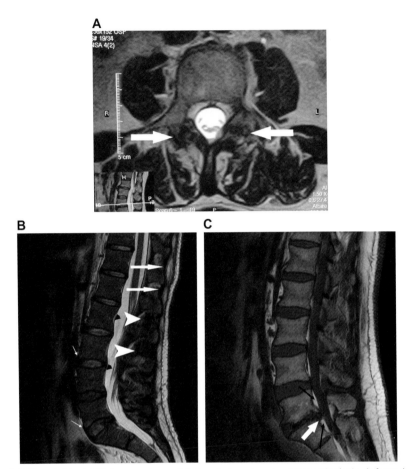

Fig. 2. (*A*) Axial T2-weighted MR image shows bilateral chronic pars interarticularis defects (*white arrows*). (*B*) Sagittal T2-weighted image shows normal interspinous (*arrowheads*) and supraspinous (*large white arrows*) ligaments, components of the posterior ligamentous complex. The ALL (*small white arrows*) is closely attached to the vertebral bodies and anterior intervertebral discs and is difficult to define. The PLL (*black arrowheads*) is less closely attached to the posterior portion of the vertebral bodies and intervertebral disc just lateral to mid-line, and is often easier to define. (*C*) Sagittal T1-weighted image shows caudal migration of a herniated disc fragment (*white arrow*) along the anterior epidural space at the L5–S1 level. Epidural fat is seen superior and inferior to the disc fragment (*black arrows*).

(grade 4b). The morphologic findings seen on cross-sectional imaging examinations can be combined with the physiologic information gathered from a single photon emission CT (SPECT) scan. Increased uptake on the SPECT scan is indicative of a pars interarticularis fracture or severe degenerative changes in this region. A classification or grading system using this combined data has been developed. According to this system, grade 0 and grade 1 changes are consistent with a normal pars or a stress reaction in this region, respectively. Grade 2 changes represent an incomplete fracture, and grades 3 and 4 represent complete fractures (acute fracture with grade 3 and chronic fracture with grade 4).

Determining the relative size of the central canal can help differentiate between the two basic types of spondylolisthesis. When the pars interarticularis is intact (degenerative spondylolisthesis), the central canal narrows, caused by the pinching effect when the vertebrae slips forward relative to the adjacent vertebral level. The instability is usually further exacerbated by hypertrophic degenerative disease at the facet joint.

The other type of spondylolisthesis, spondylolytic, has bilateral pars interarticularis defects and resultant widening of the central canal caused by anterior displacement of the arch elements anterior to the pars defects relative to the posterior portion of the neural arch. The posterior portion of the neural arch remains detached from the anterior portion because of the bony pars defects, and the result is a widening of the central canal. In spondylolytic spondylolisthesis, it is important to remember that, although the central canal becomes wider, lateral recess stenosis can develop because of the presence of callus [2]. It is also important not to mistake a sclerotic, but intact, pars for spondylolysis.

In the absence of a fracture or spondylolisthesis, vertebral malalignment can also potentially be the result of isolated ligamentous injury. As part of an alignment assessment of the spine, the anterior and posterior longitudinal ligaments (ALL and PLL, respectively) and components of the posterior ligamentous complex (which is composed of the interspinous and supraspinous ligaments and facet joint capsules) should be examined for evidence of injury (Fig. 2B).

These ligaments as a whole are best viewed using a sagittal, fluid-sensitive sequence (STIR or T2-weighted sequence with fat-saturation). Regarding the longitudinal ligaments, they should be tightly apposed to the adjacent intervertebral discs (specifically the outer annulus fibrosis). The lateral margins of the PLL are not directly attached to the posterior portion of the intervertebral disc and create a space between the PLL and the intervertebral disc. This space is the anterior epidural space and may be occupied by disc extrusions or disc fragments as they become lodged between the PLL and the disc from which they originated (Fig. 2C). Posterior disc herniation can obviously also cause focal PLL displacement, but the presence of focal ligament discontinuity (sometimes associated with adjacent soft tissue edema/hemorrhage or vertebral malalignment) is a sign of a ligament tear or perforation [3]. In the setting of acute trauma, areas of increased signal and thickening of the PLL can be seen with partial-thickness tears. Uninjured ligaments demonstrate complete signal void and are thin and linear. Normal vertebral alignment of the lumbar spine is characterized by a gentle lordotic curvature.

Evaluation of marrow-containing structures

The marrow-containing structures should be evaluated for the appropriate signal characteristics. These signal characteristics vary according to the amount of blood-producing elements, as compared with the amount of marrow fat. Usually, older patients have a relatively homogeneous-appearing, adipocyte-rich marrow, with occasional scattered areas of heterogeneity caused by the presence of more cellular hematopoietic marrow (Fig. 3A, B) [4,5].

After examining the vertebral body, one should remember to examine all other parts of the vertebrae, including the pedicles, lamina, superior and inferior articular processes, and transverse and spinous processes. This assessment should include a survey to detect any focal lesions. Common benign lesions encountered include vertebral hemangiomas (that characteristically show high T1 signal equivalent to, or higher than, adjacent bone marrow and high T2 signal) (Fig. 3C, D) [6] and bone islands, which show decreased signal on all pulse sequences and characteristic brush-border margins not always seen on MR imaging.

One should also be able to recognize a normal variant known as the limbus vertebra. The limbus vertebral body results from a separation of a triangular segment of the vertebral body ring apophysis (Fig. 3E), which may be posttraumatic or developmental and can involve the anterior or posterior vertebral body rim. This normal variant is often seen in patients who have had Scheuermann's disease. Patients who have Scheuermann's disease may also have Schmorl's nodes, intravertebral herniations commonly seen on MR imaging examinations. They have a typical appearance on cross-sectional imaging, with disc material projecting into the vertebral body through a defect in the associated end plate.

Multiple lesions that do not meet the criteria for a multifocal benign process should raise the question of metastatic disease or multiple myeloma. Increasing amounts of red marrow (manifested as decreased signal on T1-weighted images and increased signal on T2-weighted images) may be seen with failure of marrow conversion (from red marrow to yellow marrow) or in red marrow reconversion (from yellow marrow to red marrow) and can be seen in anemic states such as anemia of chronic illness, sickle cell anemia, and thalassemia (Fig. 3F).

Finally, one should check for any evidence of a marrow infiltrative process (ie, leukemia, lymphoma, Gaucher's disease, eosinophilic granuloma, or a mucopolysaccharidosis) or if myeloid depletion, where fat cells replace hematopoietic elements (as seen in aplastic anemia, radiation therapy, and chemotherapy).

The pedicles and pars interarticularis regions, in particular, should be assessed for involvement by neoplasm or fracture. MR imaging has an advantage over CT in evaluating the cancellous portion of the bone in that it can show edema within the bone itself, which may be secondary to a stress-related injury that typically precedes a frank pars interarticularis fracture [7]. This early discovery can potentially lead to earlier intervention.

In addition to assessing the pedicle for tumor involvement, the pedicles can be quickly assessed on coronal images (if they are available) and on axial views for interpediculate narrowing. This type of narrowing is usually noted on the axial images in cases of achondroplasia where the transverse interpediculate distance is decreased, and on the sagittal images in patients who have congenitally short

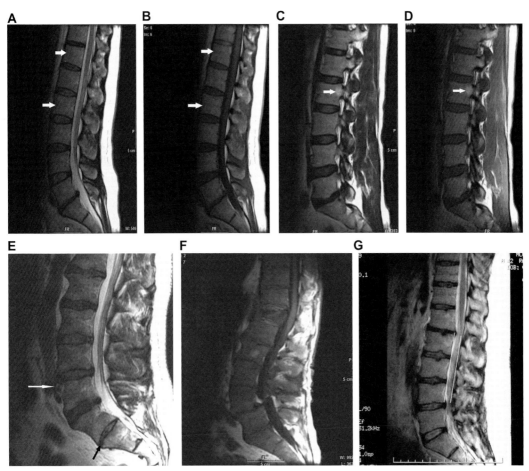

Fig. 3. (*A* and *B*) Sagittal T2-weighted and T1 images from an elderly person show patchy, heterogeneous marrow signal largely caused by adipocyte rich marrow, with scattered areas of more cellular hematopoietic marrow (*arrows*). (*C* and *D*) Sagittal T2-weighted and T1-weighted MR images show an incidental posterior L2 vertebral body hemangioma (*white arrows*), demonstrating classic increased signal on the T1- and T2-weighted images. (*E*) Sagittal T2-weighted MR image shows a limbus vertebra with a small, well-corticated, marrow-containing process (*white arrow*) representing a separation of a triangular segment of the vertebral body ring apophysis at the anterosuperior margin of L5. Note the transitional lumbosacral anatomy with a well-formed intervertebral disc at S1–S2 (*black arrow*). (*F*) Sagittal T1-weighted image shows abnormally decreased marrow signal intensity throughout the visualized spine, consistent with the presence of red marrow. (*G*) Sagittal T2-weighted image shows congenital narrowing of the spinal canal. This narrow spinal canal is decreased in size in an anterior-to-posterior dimension (*white lines*). The canal should widen slightly as it progresses from superior to inferior. This narrowing causes stenosis of the central canal and results from congenitally short pedicles.

pedicles (in the anteroposterior dimension). Narrowing of the interpediculate distance is important to note in both the anteroposterior and mediolateral dimensions because a decrease in this distance is consistent with the diagnosis of developmental or congenital spinal canal stenosis (in contradistinction to degenerative central stenosis, which will be discussed later) (Fig. 3G) [2]. Any pedicle enlargement should immediately cause the imager to consider the possibility of Paget's disease. The enlargement of the pedicles may result in lateral recess or neural foraminal stenosis.

Finally, the presence of bone marrow edema is a clue to the presence of trauma, ischemia, infection, or adjacent neoplasm. If none of these are present, idiopathic edema should then be considered. An example of normal marrow for patient age is demonstrated in Fig. 1.

Assessment of the three Cs

The imager should also assess the three Cs in sequence: cord, conus medullaris, and cauda equina nerve roots. An accurate evaluation of these structures ensures the absence of a mass or other abnormality of signal, structure size, or morphology.

The conus medullaris should be evaluated to assess for signs of tethering (eg, low-lying tip of conus medullaris below the L1–2 disc space or a thick filum terminale that is more than 2 mm in diameter). The normal cauda equina is a bundle of thin, linear, and smoothly marginated nerve roots that are present below the conus medullaris. Each nerve root should travel individually, coursing in an anterior-diagonal direction (on the sagittal images) across the central canal before entering the neural foramina. Clumping, or adherence, of nerve roots should raise suspicion for arachnoiditis. The normal appearances of the distal spinal cord, conus medullaris, and cauda equina nerve roots are shown in Fig. 4A, B.

Examination of joints, central canal, and lateral recesses

The joints, central canal, and lateral recesses should also be examined carefully, including an assessment of the degeneration-prone diarthrodial facet joints of the posterior column (of which there are two per each level) and the amphiarthrodial discovertebral joints (the end-plate–disc–end-plate joint of the anterior column). The facet joints and the discovertebral joints compose what is known as the three-joint complex of the intervertebral joint.

The normal facet joint should resemble any other normal diarthrodial joint, should demonstrate smooth cortical margins and smooth uniform articular cartilage, and should not have any significant amount of fluid or osseous proliferation.

The normal ligamentum flavum is thin and low in signal. When the ligamentum flavum is normal, it is a relatively inconspicuous-appearing structure located along the inner margins of the lamina. Degenerative thickening involving this complex is one of the primary causes of central canal and lateral recess stenosis (Fig. 5A).

An optimal way to examine the three-joint complex is to begin the assessment in the sagittal plane and then continue into the axial plane. Hypertrophic degenerative changes of the facet joints may cause central and lateral canal stenosis (Fig. 5B).

If a cystic structure is seen near a facet, it is often a degenerative facet joint cyst (Fig. 5C). After a facet joint is noted, the next point of evaluation is to determine any impingement of the cyst on the surrounding neural elements. A quantitative assessment of the amount of facet degeneration (mild, moderate, severe) should also be reported. Symptoms produced by neural impingement from a facet joint cyst can mimic the symptoms produced by a disc herniation. Correlating the presence and location of the facet cyst determines whether the facet joint cyst could be the source of the patient's symptoms. This information can be helpful in directing further therapy (ie, facet cyst aspiration, fenestration, or surgical removal) [8].

Arguably, the most important portion of the MR imaging examination interpretation is the evaluation of the discovertebral joint. The sagittal plane is optimal for showing early signs of disc disease (Fig. 5D). These early signs may include loss of

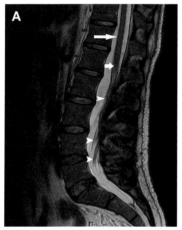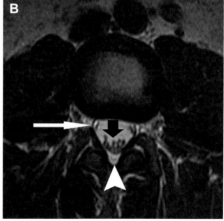

Fig. 4. (*A*) Normal MR appearance of the distal spinal cord (*long arrow*), conus medullaris (*short arrow*), and cauda equina (*arrowheads*). (*B*) Axial T2-weighted MR image of the lumbar spine shows normal soft tissues of the central canal. The fat-containing posterior epidural space is well visualized (*arrowhead*). The right lateral margin of the thecal sac is designated by a white arrow. Note the normal symmetric appearance of the cauda equina nerve roots (*black arrow*).

fluid signal within the nucleus pulposis and increasing collagen content, which results in decreased signal within the central portion of the disc, as seen on the T2-weighted images. Another early sign of degenerative disc disease is blurring of the transition between the nucleus pulposis and annulus fibrosis [9], which is typically followed later by superoinferior narrowing of the intervertebral disc.

Disc height loss and end plate/subchondral osseous changes can sometimes result in a destructive appearance, with underlying degenerative end plate changes known as Modic changes. It is important to comment on discs that have significant height loss and degenerative changes of the end plates because the presence of these changes may correlate with less than ideal outcomes when treating these patients with such techniques as percutaneous disc decompression or artificial disc replacement. Patients who have degenerative disc disease and degenerative end plate changes may be more likely to benefit from interbody fusion [8].

It is also important to know the difference between the three types of Modic degenerative end plate changes. Type I changes are characterized by signal changes of edema that are intermediate on the T1-weighted images and have increased signal on the T2-weighted images (Fig. 5E). Type II changes follow the signal characteristics of fat (Fig. 5F), and Type III changes represent bony sclerosis, characterized by decreased signal on both the T1 and T2-weighted images.

When the disc becomes degenerated or acutely injured, it may undergo tearing of the annulus fibrosis. Annular tearing represents a tear of the collagenous bundles that surround the inner nucleus pulposis. Annular tearing is part of the spectrum of intervertebral disc herniation and is often a precursor to herniation of the nucleus pulposis (Fig. 5G). The posterolateral portion of the annulus fibrosis should be closely scrutinized because this region is commonly affected by annular tearing. This tearing and disruption of the annulus fibrosis may allow for nerve ingrowth, thought to be a source of back pain because of the presence of nociceptive receptors on these nerves [10]. Circumferential or transverse annular tears should be reported but are not often associated with clinical symptoms and may just be an incidental finding. It is usually the radial-type annular tears that cause pain.

Occasionally, severe degenerative disc disease can resemble infection, and the differentiation of degenerative disc disease from spondylodiscitis often is made clinically, rather than based on the MR imaging findings. However, some MR imaging signs are more suggestive of infection than spondylosis. These findings include paravertebral soft tissue masses (such as a phlegmon or an abscess) and fluid within the intervertebral disc. Whether the underlying process is infectious or degenerative in cause, the same question must be answered: Is there significant central canal or lateral stenosis related to extension of infectious (or degenerative) material into the epidural space?

A useful imaging method that can be applied to the detection of spinal stenosis is to look for the trefoil. A trefoil shape is a somewhat triangular shape that is indicative of central canal stenosis in the lumbar spine, and is typically the result of ligamentum flavum hypertrophy and intervertebral disc bulging or herniation (Fig. 5H). Posterior end plate osteophytes or facet joint degenerative disease may also contribute to this appearance of the spinal canal. Although the authors do not discuss the differences among the various types and locations of disc herniations (ie, bulge versus protrusion versus extrusion and the resulting central/lateral recess/foraminal stenosis), it is imperative that all physicians involved in the interpretation of spinal imaging studies communicate using the same terminology. Standard descriptive nomenclature for describing lumbar spine intervertebral disc herniations was introduced in 2001 when a combined task force from the North American Spine Society, the American Society of Spine Radiology, and the American Society of Neuroradiology documented a standard nomenclature and classification system [11].

Although degenerative causes of central canal narrowing at the disc level include bulging or herniated discs, the most common causes of spinal canal narrowing are hypertrophy of the ligamentum flavum, spondylolisthesis, and displacement of facet joints. Other processes, such as postoperative or posttraumatic changes, malignancy, Paget's disease, and synovial cysts, may also contribute to narrowing of the spinal canal.

Impingement of the nerves as they course from the central portion of the spinal canal to the lumbosacral plexus is a common cause of discomfort and is often seen in patients who have low back pain and radicular symptoms. The nerves may be impinged on at any point along this course, and appropriate knowledge of the anatomy of the course of the nerve root assists in the detection of pathology that may result in nerve root impingement. If the lumbar spine MR imaging examination includes a coronal plane (many institutions forego the coronal plane in routine MR imaging of the lumbar spine but include it in the evaluation of patients who have scoliosis), one should be able to appreciate the three described zones of lateral stenosis. If no coronal plane is available, the axial plane may be used to estimate the zone of nerve impingement. Zone I includes the lateral recess (or entrance zone) and is medial or central to the pedicle. The lateral margin of zone I is the medial cortical margin of the pedicle. Zone II (also known as the neural foramen) is strictly the space between the pedicles, and zone III (the exit zone) is the portion of the foramen proper that is outside the canal (Fig. 5I–L) [12]. The lateral recess can be narrowed from an anterior pathologic process, most commonly a disc herniation, or from a posterolateral/inferior pathologic process such as hypertrophic facet arthrosis (the inferior portion of the recess is bordered inferiorly by the superior facet from the vertebrae below). Zone II is prone to narrowing by movements in the facet joint and by hypertrophic facet joint arthrosis. Zone III is typically narrowed with a far lateral disc herniation.

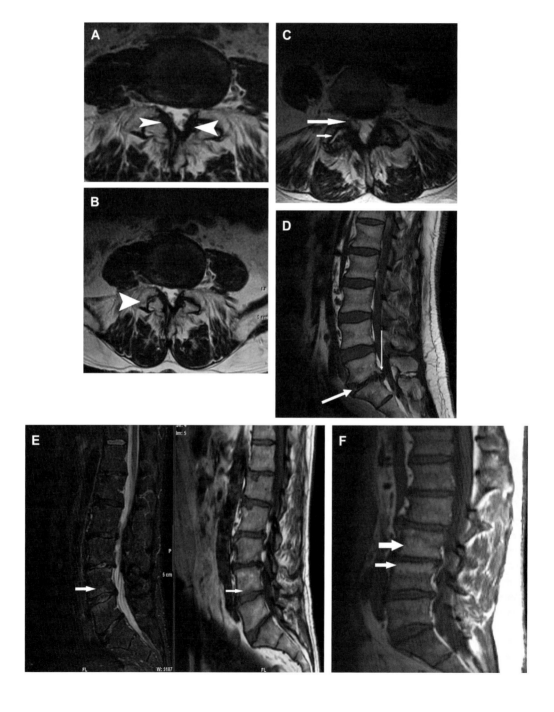

Finally, a level-by-level reporting of central and lateral canal stenosis and any associated neural compromise is useful to communicate this information clearly and concisely. It may be reported as follows:

T12–L1: (This level almost always normal.)

L1–L2: (This level is often normal.)

L2–L3: (Mild degenerative changes are often seen at this level.)

L3–L4: (More severe degenerative disease typically begins at this level.)

L4–L5: (This level is commonly affected by more severe degenerative disease.)

L5–S1: (This level often demonstrates the most severe intervertebral osteochondrosis, but neural compromise is less common than at the L4–L5 level.)

Spondylotic anterior osteophyte formation caused by traction on the ALL and perivertebral ligaments is ubiquitous and deserves only very brief mention here and in the imaging report, unless the degree of spondylosis is out of proportion to what would be expected for the patient's age. Spondylosis is extremely common and is a normal component of the aging spine. In addition to noting spondylotic change that is out of proportion to what would be expected for the patient's age, it is important to note any significant mass effect that the osteophytes have on soft tissue structures anterior to them. Spondylosis should also be differentiated from syndesmophytes, which represent the ossification of the annulus fibrosis of the intervertebral discs and are usually indicative of a different disease process.

◄ ───

Fig. 5. (A) Axial T2-weighted MR image demonstrates degenerative thickening and irregularity of the ligamentum flavum (*arrowheads*). Hypertrophy of the ligamentum flavum narrows the posterior portion of the spinal canal and contributes to acquired central canal stenosis. (B) Axial T2-weighted MR image of the lumbar spine shows hypertrophic degenerative facet joints (*arrowhead indicates right facet joint*). These hypertrophic degenerative changes may contribute to lateral and central spinal canal narrowing. (C) Axial T2-weighted MR image shows a region of increased signal just anteromedial to the right facet joint (*large white arrow*), which is consistent with a facet joint cyst, and this cyst is causing encroachment of the central canal and lateral recess. Note the presence of ipsilateral facet joint fluid (*small white arrow*). This fluid represents a small facet joint effusion. (D) Sagittal T1-weighted MR image shows severe degenerative disc disease at the L5–S1 level (*thick white arrow*). An associated posterior disc herniation and a disc/osteophyte complex at the L5–S1 level (*thin white arrow*) may also be noted. The remainder of the lumbar spine intervertebral discs are relatively preserved. (E) Sagittal T2-weighted (*left*) and T1-weighted (*right*) MR images showing type I Modic degenerative end plate changes. Type I changes are seen as edema within the bone marrow immediately subjacent to the end plate of the intervertebral disc. This edema is seen as increased signal on the T2-weighted images (*white arrow on the T2-weighted MR image on the left*) and intermediate-to-decreased signal on the T1-weighted image (*white arrow on the T1-weighted MR image on the right*). (F) Sagittal T1-weighted MR image demonstrates type II Modic degenerative end plate changes (*white arrows*), which follow the signal characteristics of fat on all pulse sequences. The degenerative end plate signal changes are slightly more extensive in the inferior portion of the L3 vertebral body (*thicker white arrow*) than in the adjacent superior portion of the L4 vertebral body (*thinner white arrow*). (G) Sagittal T2-weighted MR image shows focal high signal intensities in the posterior portions of the L4–5 and L5–S1 intervertebral discs. These focal regions of increased signal are consistent with a circumferential annular tear at both the L4–5 and L5–S1 levels (*white arrows*). Annular tears such as these may or may not be symptomatic. Note the loss of distinction between the nucleus pulposus and the annulus fibrosis (*short black arrows*), which reflects the loss of hydration within the nucleus pulposis. (H) Axial T2-weighted MR image through the midlumbar spine shows ligamentum flavum thickening (*small white arrowhead*) and hypertrophic degenerative facet joint disease (*long larger white arrows*). A very small amount of fluid within the right facet joint space is also shown (*smaller white arrow*). These degenerative changes, in conjunction with the broad-based disc bulge (*large white arrowheads*), result in a moderately narrowed central canal at this level. Note that the shape of the narrowed central canal (*white dotted line*) has been described as a trefoil shape. (I) Sagittal (*left*) and axial (*right*) T2-weighted MR images show the anatomic location of zone I of the nerve root pathway (*white crosshair on both the sagittal and axial images*). Zone I includes the lateral recess (or entrance zone) and is medial or central to the corresponding pedicle. (J) Sagittal (*left*) and axial (*right*) T2-weighted MR images show the anatomic location of zone II of the nerve root pathway (also known as the neural foramen). (Zone II is indicated by white crosshair on both the sagittal and axial images). This zone is defined as the space between the pedicles. (K) Sagittal T2-weighted MR image of the right neural foramen shows the dorsal nerve root ganglion (*smaller white arrow pointing posteriorly*) located in the superior portion of the neural foramen. Small vessels (*larger white arrow pointing anteriorly*) are seen coursing toward the inferior recess of the spinal neural foramen (*white arrowhead*). (L) Sagittal (*left*) and axial (*right*) T2-weighted MR images show the anatomic location of zone III (the exit zone). (Zone III is indicated by the white crosshairs.) This portion of the neural foramen proper is located outside of the canal.

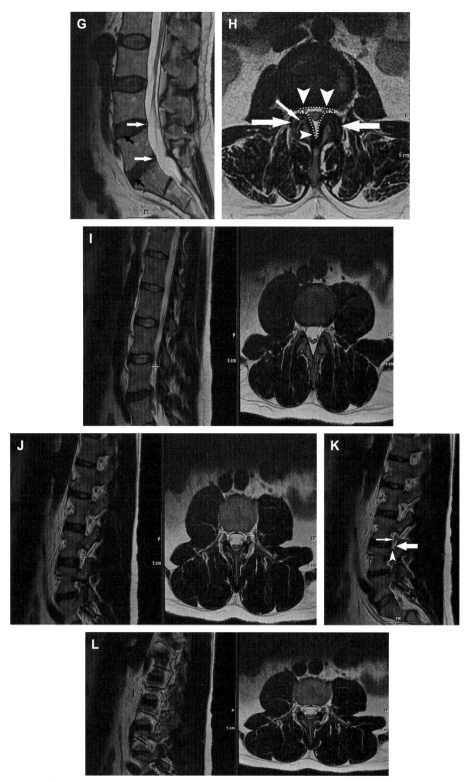

Fig. 5 (continued).

Examination of paravertebral soft tissues and other osseous elements

Finally, the imager should examine the paravertebral soft tissues and other osseous elements. The visualized retroperitoneal soft tissues (including the aorta, kidneys, and psoas muscles) should be looked at on the axial images. Renal cysts and hydronephrosis are commonly seen and the adrenal glands are often imaged on the axial portion of the MR imaging examination. A psoas abscess can be seen with spondylodiscitis, renal tumors may be noted on the axial images, and any process affecting the retroperitoneum may be detected by closely examining the retroperitoneal soft tissues. The sacrum and sacroiliac joints are also imaged to various degrees and these areas deserve a quick look to exclude significant unsuspected pathology, such as sacral insufficiency fractures or sacroiliitis. Degenerative disease in these regions is very common and should be noted as part of the overall assessment.

A final cautionary note is that all abnormal MR imaging findings need clinical correlation because it has been shown that many asymptomatic patients can have abnormal MR imaging examination findings [13]. Although cartilage, tendon, or ligamentous abnormalities in the knee and shoulder are usually symptomatic in these regions, anatomic abnormalities in the lumbar spine may not necessarily be symptomatic, or areas that demonstrate more subtle anatomic abnormalities may cause more symptoms than the more obvious anatomic derangements. Routine lumbar spine MR imaging examinations are also limited in that they currently image in a static manner with relatively neutral supine positioning (and without provocative movements). Neural foraminal and spinal canal stenosis can be seen frequently in extension and flexion, rotation, and lateral bending to a greater degree than in the conventional neutral imaging position [14].

Summary

The systematic approach to lumbar spine MR imaging examination interpretation may therefore be summarized as follows:

1. General overview
2. Spinal alignment/ligaments
3. Marrow-containing structures
4. The 3 Cs: cord, conus, cauda equina
5. Joints and the canal (both central and lateral canals)
6. Other (retroperitoneal soft tissues, sacrum, sacroiliac joints)
7. Concise diagnostic impression (rendered while recognizing that the clinician will need to correlate the MR imaging findings with the patient's clinical symptoms and physical examination findings)

This approach is just one of a multitude of possible approaches to assessing the anatomic status of the lumbar spine. It may be used as presented, or altered for more specific needs or according to each individual reader. Once the approach is established, one should avoid deviating from the standard approach because repetition and the thoroughness associated with following a comprehensive systematic approach will undoubtedly contribute to increased efficiency and accuracy of the diagnostic interpretation.

References

[1] Campbell RSD, Grainger AJ, Hide IG, et al. Juvenile spondylolysis: a comparative analysis of CT, SPECT and MRI. Skeletal Radiol 2005;34:63–73.
[2] Schonstrom N, Willen J. Imaging lumbar spinal stenosis. Radiol Clin North Am 2001;39:31–53.
[3] Pathria M. Imaging of spine instability. Semin Musculoskelet Radiol 2005;9:88–99.
[4] Vande Berg BC, Malghem J, Lecouvet FE, et al. Magnetic resonance imaging of the normal bone marrow. Skeletal Radiol 1998;27:471–83.
[5] Vogler JB, Murphy WA. Bone marrow imaging. Radiology 1988;168:679–93.
[6] Ross JS, Masaryk TJ, Modic MT, et al. Vertebral hemangiomas: MR imaging. Radiology 1987; 165:165–9.
[7] Hollenburg GM, Beattie PF, Meyers SP, et al. Stress reactions of the lumbar pars interarticularis: the development of a new MRI classification system. Spine 2002;27:181–6.
[8] Thalgott JS, Albert TJ, Vaccaro AR, et al. A new classification system for degenerative disc disease of the lumbar spine based on magnetic resonance imaging, provocative discography, plain radiographs and anatomic considerations. Spine J 2004;4(6 Suppl):167S–72S.
[9] Eisenstein S, Roberts S. The physiology of the disc and its clinical relevance. J Bone Joint Surg Br 2003;85:633–6.
[10] Yoshizawa H, O'Brien JP, Smith WT, et al. The neuropathology of intervertebral discs removed for low-back pain. J Pathol 1980;132(2):95–104.
[11] Fardon DF, Milette PC, Combined task forces of the North American Spine society, American Society of Spine Radiology, and American Society of Neuroradiology. Nomenclature and classification of lumbar disc pathology. Recommendations of the combined task forces of the North American Spine Society, American Society of Spine Radiology, and American Society of Neuroradiology. Spine 2001;26:E93–113.

[12] Anderson GBJ, McNeill TW. Lumbar spine syndromes. Vienna (Austria): Springer-Verlag; 1989.

[13] Borenstein DG, O'Mara JW Jr, Boden SD, et al. The value of magnetic resonance imaging of the lumbar spine to predict low-back pain in asymptomatic subjects: a seven-year follow-up study. J Bone Joint Surg Am 2001; 83:1306–11.

[14] Nowicki BH, Haughton VM, Schmidt TA, et al. Occult lumbar lateral spinal stenosis in neural foramina subjected to physiologic loading. AJNR Am J Neuroradiol 1996;17:1605–14.

MAGNETIC
RESONANCE
IMAGING CLINICS

Magn Reson Imaging Clin N Am 15 (2007) 167–174

Nomenclature and Standard Reporting Terminology of Intervertebral Disk Herniation

Richard F. Costello, DO[a],*, Douglas P. Beall, MD[a,b]

- Discussion
- Summary
- References

Anatomic derangement of the spine is extremely common and may be seen in symptomatic and asymptomatic individuals. The terminology used to describe intervertebral disk herniations is complex and many of the common references differ in their nomenclature used to report disk pathology. The nomenclature contained in this article is based on recommendations from The North American Spine Society, The American Society of Neuroradiology, and The American Society of Spine Radiology [1].

The intent of the recommendations are to standardize the reporting of the size and location of intervertebral disk lesions and to simplify the anatomic descriptions of findings on CT and MR imaging. Recommendations are to report abnormalities in zones on axial images and in levels on the sagittal and coronal images. The size of the herniation may be described in words or numbers. The terminology may be used in the cervical and thoracic spine, but was primarily developed for use in the lumbar spine.

Discussion

There are 23 intervertebral disks between adjacent vertebral bodies from C2 to S1. The disks are thicker anteriorly in the cervical and lumbar spine, which contributes to the lordosis normally seen in these regions of the spine. In the thoracic spine the intervertebral disks are uniform in thickness. The intervertebral disks contribute approximately one fourth of the length to the vertebral column.

The normal intervertebral disk has an inner nucleus pulposus and an outer annulus fibrosus and is bordered by the cartilage end plates (Fig. 1). The nucleus pulposus contains hydrophilic glycosaminoglycans with a lattice of collagen fibers. Over time the gelatinous glycosaminoglycans is replaced by fibrocartilage [2]. The annulus fibrosus contains 15 to 20 collagenous laminae that are organized obliquely to one another and are weakest posterolaterally where the collagen bundles are less organized. The cartilage end plates are composed of hyaline cartilage and are the anatomic limit of the disk with the posterior portion of disk forming part of the anterior wall of the neural foramen. The intervertebral disc is avascular and aneural and obtains its nutrition by diffusion from the adjacent vertebral body and end plates.

An annular tear is a concentric, radial, or transverse separation of the annular fibers. Annular tears (Fig. 2) can be found in a minority of individuals over 40 years of age and are considered

a Clinical Radiology of Oklahoma, 610 NW 14th Street, Oklahoma City, OK 73103, USA
b University of Oklahoma, 610 NW 14th Street, Oklahoma City, OK 73103, USA
* Corresponding author.
E-mail address: ecostellodo@okss.com (R.F. Costello).

1064-9689/07/$ – see front matter © 2007 Elsevier Inc. All rights reserved.
mri.theclinics.com

doi:10.1016/j.mric.2006.12.001

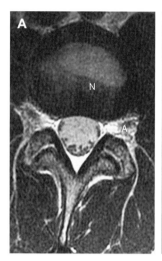
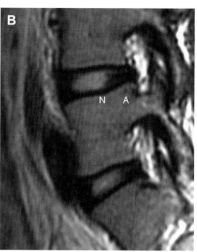

Fig. 1. Axial (*A*) and sagittal (*B*) T2-weighted MR images demonstrate the increased signal of the normal nucleus pulposus (N) and decreased signal of the normal annulus fibrosis (A).

pathologic and a precursor to intervertebral disk herniation. Most annular tears are not visible on MR imaging, but those tears that are visible demonstrate a high intensity zone that is often crescent shaped and is commonly seen in the posterior portion of the disk at L4-5 and L5-S1. Radial tears demonstrate disruption perpendicular to the axis of the collagen fibers. The disruption extends from the gelatinous nucleus pulposus through the annulus fibrosis to the periphery of the disk and may be painful, especially if the tear is located immediately adjacent to the dorsal nerve root ganglion. The dorsal nerve root ganglion gives rise to the sinuvertebral nerve that innervates the posterolateral portion of the intervertebral disk. Tears of the annulus fibrosis to the periphery of the disk also allow nerve and granulation tissue ingrowth into the disk. Concentric tears are disruption parallel to the axis of the collagen fibers. This forms

a high intensity zone between adjacent collagen fibers. The significance of an annular tear is controversial and the presence may not correlate with the need for treatment or with clinical symptoms [3].

Herniation is the term used most commonly to describe the displacement of disk material. This can involve displacement of the nucleus pulposus, end plate cartilage, fragmented apophyseal bone, or annular tissue beyond the normal confines of the disk space. Intervertebral disk herniations may occur centrifugally out from the periphery of the disk or in a superior or inferior direction. A disk herniation is a localized (involving less than 50% of the circumference of the disk or less than 180° of the periphery of the disk) displacement of disk material beyond the normal confines of the disk. This is in contrast to a disk bulge that involves more than half of the circumference (more than

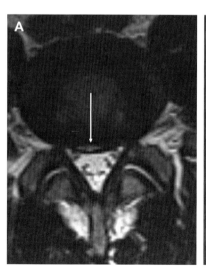
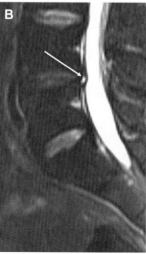

Fig. 2. Axial (*A*) and sagittal (*B*) T2-weighted MR images demonstrate a crescentic area (*arrows*) of increased signal (high intensity zone) in the posterior portion of the disk at L4-5. This is characteristic appearance of an annular tear.

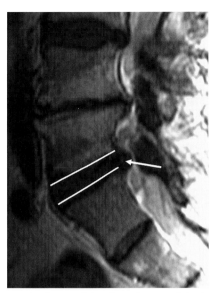

Fig. 3. Sagittal T2-weighted MR image of the lumbar spine demonstrates a disk protrusion at the L5-S1 level (*white arrow*). Note that the protruded disk material does not extend beyond the confines of the superior and inferior disk borders (ie, beyond the disk/end plate junction). As defined on the sagittal plane, this disk herniation may be described as a protrusion.

180° of the disk) or the entire disk. Herniation is a general term that can be further characterized as a protrusion or extrusion based on the shape and amount of the displaced disk material [4].

A herniated disk is a protrusion if the greatest distance of the edges of the protruded material is less than the edges of the normal disk material as determined on the same plane. For example, if the greatest superoinferior distance of the edges of the herniated disk material is less than or equal to the edges of the normal disk in the same plane (as measured on the sagittal or coronal plane to assess superoinferior extension), then this is classified as a disk protrusion (Fig. 3). The superoinferior measurement is nearly always best determined on the sagittal plane. A protrusion, as determined on the axial plane, is a herniated portion of the disk that involves less than half of the disk (<180° of the disk circumference). Protrusions may be further classified as focal or broad, based on their degree of disk involvement. A focal protrusion involves less than 25% (or 90°) of disk circumference, whereas broad-based protrusions involve between 25% and 50% (90°–180°) of the disk circumference (Fig. 4).

In contrast to a protrusion, a herniated disk is an extrusion if the greatest distance of the edges of the herniated material is greater than the distance between the edges of the base of the herniation as measured on the same plane. For example, if disk material is displaced beyond the confines of the superior or inferior border of the disk or end plates as seen on the sagittal plane, this would constitute a disk extrusion (Fig. 5). If the extruded disk material has a narrow neck and a wider extruded portion as seen on the axial plane, this would also be best described as a disk extrusion (Fig. 6). In contrast, a protrusion would not extend beyond the superior or inferior border of the intervertebral disk on the sagittal images and would have a broad-based neck with a protruded portion of the disk that was not as wide as the neck of the protrusion (see Figs. 5 and 6).

Disk extrusions may be further classified into sequestrations or migrated disks. A migrated disk is a disk or disk fragment that has been displaced

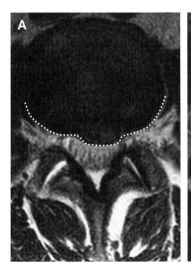
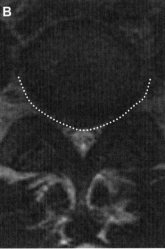

Fig. 4. Axial T2-weighted MR images taken through the L4-5 intervertebral disk show disk protrusions. Focal (*A*) and broad-based disk (*B*) protrusions are outlined by the dotted white line. A focal protrusion involves less than 25% (or 90°) of disk circumference, whereas broad-based protrusions involve between 25% and 50% (90°–180°) of the disk circumference.

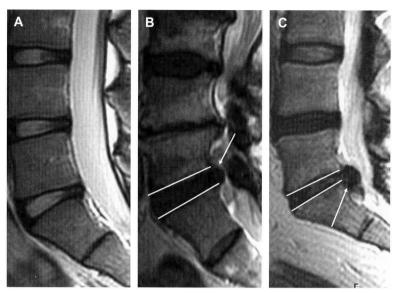

Fig. 5. Sagittal MR images of the lumbar spine demonstrate normal intervertebral discs (*A*), a disk protrusion at L5-S1 (*arrow*) (*B*), disk extrusion with inferior displacement at L5-S1 (*arrow*) (*C*). The superior and inferior borders of the L5-S1 intervertebral disks are indicated by the solid white lines in *B* and *C*. Protrusions do not extend beyond the superoinferior dimension of the disk in the sagittal plane (*B*), whereas extrusions extend beyond this border (*C*).

away from the site of the extrusion but still retains continuity with the disk from which the extrusion originated. Sequestrations are disk extrusions that become detached from the parent disk (Fig. 7). Describing sequestrations are important, because a sequestered disk may be a contraindication to minimally invasive therapies such as a microdiskectomies, percutaneous radio frequency ablations, percutaneous mechanical disk decompression, or the use of intradiscal steroids.

Intervertebral disk herniations may also be categorized according to the degree of containment. Containment refers to the status of the annular fibers that surround the nucleus pulposis. If the outer annulus is intact, the disk herniation would be classified as contained and would not have any type of communication with the epidural space or spinal canal. If iodinated contrast is injected into a contained herniation, for example, it will not leak into the epidural space or the spinal canal from

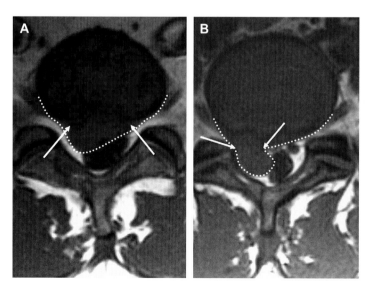

Fig. 6. Axial T1-weighted MR images of the lumbar spine at the L4-5 level show posterior disk herniations. (*A*) The herniation (*white dotted line*) shows a wider neck (*white arrows*); (*B*) herniation (*white dotted line*) shows a narrow neck (*white arrows*).

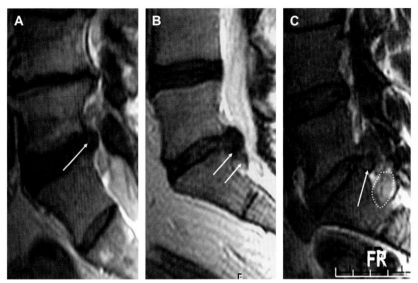

Fig. 7. Sagittal T2-weighted MR images of the lumbar spine demonstrate a disk protrusion (*white arrow*) (*A*). Note that the superoinferior extent of the protruded disk does not extend superior or inferior to the respective endplates. A disk extrusion with inferior extension of disk material beyond the confines of the superior endplate of S1 (*white arrows*) (*B*). A disk extrusion with inferior migration of the intervertebral disk beyond the confines of the superior endplate of S1 (*white arrow*) (*C*). A disk fragment (sequestered disk fragment) is also seen inferior to the disk extrusion (*white dotted line*).

a defect within the annulus fibrosis. Other descriptions of intervertebral disk herniations elucidate their relationship to the posterior longitudinal ligament (PLL). In this description scheme, various types of herniations may be categorized as subligamentous, transligamentous, or extraligamentous, depending on whether the disk herniation is ventral to the PLL, has extended through the PLL, or has herniated in a region not bounded posteriorly by the PLL, respectively (Fig. 8) [4]. Although this descriptive scheme is effective at localizing the disk herniation when the PLL is seen as a distinct

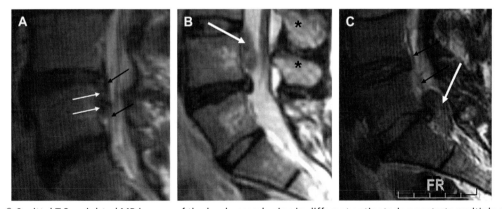

Fig. 8. Sagittal T-2 weighted MR images of the lumbosacral spine in different patients demonstrate multiple disk herniations. (*A*) The disk herniation extends inferiorly from its origin at the L4-5 intervertebral disk (*white arrows*) and is located immediately anterior to the posterior longitudinal ligament (PLL) (*black arrows*) within the anterior epidural space. (*B*) The disk extrusion (*white arrow*) is located in the midline (note the spinous processes as indicated by the *black asterisks*) and just posterior to the PLL, which is not well demonstrated on this midline image because it is directly adherent to the posterior portions of the vertebral bodies. The disk herniation was determined to have extruded into the spinal canal through the PLL (a transligamentous herniation). (*C*) A disk extrusion (*white arrow*) is seen posterior to the PLL (*black arrows*) and originated just lateral to the PLL. This may be termed an extraligamentous disk herniation.

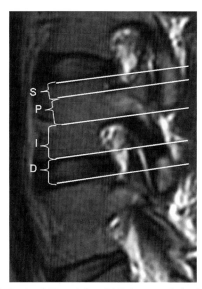

Fig. 9. Sagittal T2-weighted MR image of the lumbar spine showing the level categories of disk herniation. D, disc level; I, infrapedicular; P, pedicular; S, suprapedicular.

structure, it is difficult to distinguish the PLL from the outer fibers of the annulus fibrosis or from the dural membrane. The relationship of the disk to the PLL primarily depends upon the sagittal location of the abnormality. Centrally the PLL attaches directly to the posterior vertebral body where there is no potential space. Paracentrally the PLL narrows in its lateral extent and is not firmly attached to the posterior portion of the vertebral body thereby creating a space known as the anterior epidural space. This space is an important anatomic location to identify because disk fragments are frequently trapped within the anterior epidural space (see Fig. 8).

Location of disk herniations may be described according to various anatomic zones in the axial plane and according to various anatomic levels on the sagittal or coronal planes [5]. Herniations in the coronal and sagittal planes are defined by the craniocaudal extent of the herniation, and the description of the herniation is in comparison to the pedicle. The descriptors are suprapedicular, pedicular, infrapedicular, and disc level herniations (Figs. 9 and 10). The axial classification of disk herniation location is more pragmatic and useful because it describes the location of the herniation relative to the various exiting and traversing nerves. In the axial classification scheme, the medial edge of the facet articulations and the borders of the pedicles or the neural formina are used for anatomic landmarks. The description of the location of the herniation is not always easy because the surfaces and landmarks of the pedicles and facet joints are curved, and drawing a distinct border may be difficult or occasionally impossible. In the axial plane

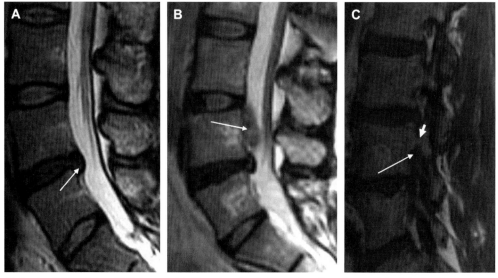

Fig. 10. Sagittal T2-weighted MR images (*A, B*) and sagittal T1-weighted MR image (*C*) of the lumbar spine shows multiple different disk herniations at various levels. (*A*) Disk herniation at L4-5 with minimal displacement of the herniation inferiorly (*white arrow*); this disk herniation is located at a suprapedicular level. (*B*) Disk extrusion originating from the L4-5 level with a sequestered disk fragment located at the level of the pedicle (*white arrow*). (*C*) Disk extrusion originating from the L4-5 level and extending superiorly to be positioned in an infrapedicular location (*white arrow*). The pedicle (*white arrowhead*) is seen just above the superior location of the disk herniation.

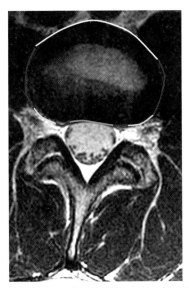

Fig. 11. Axial T2-weighted MR image taken through the L3-4 level shows the various intervertebral disk zones as defined on the axial view. The green line segment indicates the central zone, the blue line segments indicate the subarticular zones, the yellow line segments indicate the foraminal zones, the red line segments indicate the extraforaminal zones, and the white line segment indicates the anterior zone.

the boundaries or zones are defined as the central zone, the subarticular zone, the foraminal zone, the extraforaminal or far lateral zone, and the anterior zone (Fig. 11). Most disk herniations will occupy more than one zone and many will occupy more than one level.

Description of disk herniations should also be described in relation to the nerves and should communicate which nerves are involved and where they are displaced or impinged. This not only facilitates preoperative planning, but the exact location of the abnormality must be accurately described to determine whether or not the patient's clinical symptoms correspond to the location of the herniation found on the MR imaging examination. This correlation must be done in a fastidious way to avoid surgery at an incorrect spinal level. Often herniations may be multiple and patients can be symptomatic from one herniation and not another. The vast majority of disk herniations (90% or more) will occur in a central or subarticular location. When a disk herniation occurs in this location, it will most often affect the traversing nerve root (ie, a paracentral disk herniation at the L4-5 level will most often affect the traversing L5 nerve root rather than the exiting L4 nerve root) (Fig. 12). Only approximately 4% to 5% of disk herniations occur in the foraminal or extraforaminal location. These herniations are not only far less common than the paracentral disk herniations but they affect the exiting nerve roots at the levels which they occur (ie, a foraminal or extraforminal disk herniation at the L4-5 level will most often affect the exiting L4 nerve root rather than the traversing L5 nerve root) (see Fig. 12). A foraminal or extraforaminal disk herniation will therefore tend to mimic a disk herniation at one spinal level higher. Using the example above, the L4 nerve root will be more commonly affected by a central or subarticular disk herniation at the L3-4 level rather than by

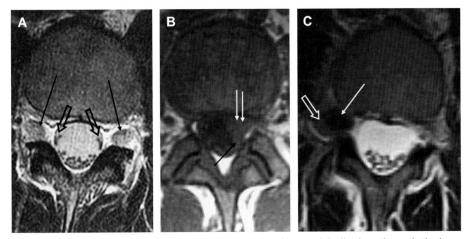

Fig. 12. Axial T2-weighted images (A, C) and an axial T1-weighted image (B) all taken through the lower lumbar spine show various findings. (A) Normal exiting nerve roots (*black arrows*) and normal traversing nerve roots (*open black arrows*). (B) A left central and subarticular disk protrusion (*white arrows*) that displaces the traversing nerve root (*black arrow*). (C) A foraminal disk herniation that displaces the exiting nerve root (*open white arrow*) posterolaterally.

a forminal or extraforminal disk herniation at the L4-5 level. Whenever the latter type of disk herniations occur, it is important to accurately identify these to prevent an unnecessary surgery at the level above (see Fig. 12).

Summary

Intervertebral disk herniation is a commonly encountered condition that may be found in both symptomatic and nonsymptomatic patients. The traditional terminology that has been used to describe the type of herniation has varied widely. The authors present standard and recommended nomenclature used to describe disk herniations for the purpose of simplifying and standardizing the reporting of the abnormalities in hopes that this will improve the accuracy of the communication of anatomic findings. A precursor to disk herniation is an annular tear that represents a linear disruption of the fibers of the annulus fibrosis. Most annular tears are not visible on MR imaging but some may be seen as a high intensity zone. Herniations may result from annular tears and may be further divided into protrusions or extrusions depending its severity. An extrusion is a more extensive herniation and may have disk material that migrates inferiorly or superiorly, may become displaced into the anterior epidural space, or may become detached as sequestered disk fragment. Herniations may also be classified according to the degree of annulus containment and to their location as it relates to the posterior longitudinal ligament. One of the most important underpinnings of the standard reporting system is the axial definition of the location of the herniation. The location defines which nerve is most likely to be affected by the herniation. It is especially important to detect the less common foraminal and extraforaminal disk herniations because these types can affect the exiting nerve root rather than the more commonly affected traversing nerve root and can mimic a paracentral disk herniation at one level above. An adequate understanding of the pathology contributing to the process of disk herniation, the category of herniation that is present, the important structures to which it relates, and how to appropriately communicate this information will contribute to a highly accurate patient assessment and will hopefully decrease the number of surgical procedures at the incorrect anatomic site.

References

[1] Fardon DF, Milette PC. Combined Task Forces of the North American Spine Society, American Society of Spine Radiology, and American Society of Neuroradiology. Nomenclature and classification of lumbar disc pathology. Recommendations of the Combined Task Forces of the North American Spine Society, American Society of Spine Radiology, and American Society of Neuroradiology. Spine 2001;26(5):E93–113.

[2] Jarvik JG, Haynor DR, Koepsell TD, et al. Interreader reliability for a new classification of lumbar disc abnormalities. Acad Radiol 1996;3:537–44.

[3] Milette PC. The proper terminology for reporting lumbar intervertebral disk disorders. AJNR Am J Neuroradiol 1997;18:1859–66.

[4] Milette PC. Classification, diagnostic imaging and imaging characterization of a lumbar herniated disc. Radiol Clin North Am 2000;38:1267–92.

[5] Wiltse LL, Berger PE, McCulloch JA. A system for reporting the size and location of lesions in the spine. Spine 1997;22(13):1534–7.

MAGNETIC
RESONANCE
IMAGING CLINICS

Magn Reson Imaging Clin N Am 15 (2007) 175–198

ELSEVIER
SAUNDERS

MR Imaging of the Spinal Bone Marrow

MAJ Michael A. Tall, MD[a],*, Adrianne K. Thompson, MD[b],
Talia Vertinsky, MD[b], COL Peter S. Palka, DO[a]

Adequate interpretation of a cervical, thoracic, or lumbar spine MR imaging examination includes a careful evaluation of the bone marrow. Detecting an abnormality in the bone marrow may cause a diagnostic dilemma because the marrow can have a variable appearance. The bone marrow in the spine can vary in appearance according to the patient's age [1], and can be affected by infectious, inflammatory, metabolic, and neoplastic processes. Its appearance can be affected as well by underlying degenerative disc disease [2], trauma, and numerous iatrogenic therapies, including vertebroplasty, radiation therapy [3], and medications designed to stimulate the bone marrow. In addition to conventional MR imaging sequences, such as T1- and T2-weighted imaging, short tau inversion recovery

(STIR), gradient echo, and contrast-enhanced imaging, newer imaging sequences, such as diffusion weighting and opposed-phase sequences, are being studied currently to help increase the diagnostic accuracy of spine and bone marrow evaluation and to help differentiate benign from malignant and infectious processes.

Anatomic and developmental considerations

The marrow is the production site of the circulating blood elements, and after 24 weeks of gestation, the marrow is the main organ of hematopoiesis. Bone marrow consists of three basic components: red marrow, yellow marrow, and trabecular bone.

[a] Department of Radiology, David Grant Medical Center, 101 Bodin Circle, Travis Air Force Base, CA 94535, USA
[b] Department of Radiology, Stanford University School of Medicine, 300 Pasteur Drive, Stanford, CA 94305, USA
* Corresponding author.
E-mail address: michael.tall@travis.af.mil (M.A. Tall).

doi:10.1016/j.mric.2007.01.001

Active areas of hematopoiesis, often referred to as red marrow, are uniformly present throughout the skeleton at birth. The function of yellow marrow is not understood completely; however, it may provide nutritional support for the hematopoietic elements. It has a limited blood supply. Trabecular bone can be thought of as providing structural support for the red and yellow marrow elements; it also stores minerals such as calcium and phosphate.

The normal distribution of marrow and, subsequently, its MR appearance, vary with age [1]. As maturation occurs, a normal physiologic conversion of active hematopoietic (or red) marrow to inactive hematopoietic (or yellow) marrow occurs in an orderly fashion, eventually establishing an adult distribution by age 25. In the adult, the hematopoietic marrow is concentrated in a central distribution within the appendicular and axial skeletons. In the spine, the presence of fatty marrow increases with advancing age.

Four patterns of physiologic conversion of active hematopoietic red marrow to fatty bone marrow in the vertebral bodies have been described with age on T1-weighted spin echo images [1]. In pattern 1, linear areas of high signal intensity parallel the basivertebral vein. The remainder of the vertebral body is uniformly low in signal intensity. The low signal intensity is attributed to the red marrow. This pattern was observed in nearly one half of those younger than 20, and in essentially no one older than 30. In pattern 2, the conversion to fatty marrow is at the periphery of the vertebral body. Along the anterior and posterior corners of the vertebral bodies and near the endplates, bandlike and triangular regions of high signal intensity are found. This pattern may be seen with degenerative disc disease. In pattern 3, diffusely distributed areas of high signal intensity are seen and described by size. Pattern 3a consists of numerous, indistinct, high signal intensity foci, measuring a few millimeters or less. Pattern 3b consists of fairly well marginated regions of high signal intensity, ranging in size from 0.5 to 1.5 cm. In those older than 40, approximately 85% show pattern 2 and approximately 75% show pattern 3. Combinations of patterns 2, 3a, and 3b may be seen in a few cases. Often, with the development of osteoporosis, fatty replacement is associated with the loss of cancellous bone and trabeculae. Under normal circumstances, the marrow is not composed entirely of either all red or all yellow marrow, but is intermixed, with different areas of the skeleton having different proportions of each, and this is what accounts for its appearance on MR imaging. Marrow reconversion is a process that occurs during times of stress, in which the body requires increased blood cell production, such as in response to anemia. It occurs in the reverse order of maturation and favors areas of residual hematopoietic sites.

Standard imaging of the spinal marrow

Standard imaging sequences include T1- and T2-weighting, with or without fat saturation, and STIR sequences. Newer imaging protocols have been developed that are useful in quantifying marrow fat (eg, for use in Gaucher's disease), as well as diffusion-weighted and opposed-phase sequences, which show promise in differentiating between various pathologic processes. Intravenous gadolinium administration is useful for assessing the paraspinal soft tissues, to distinguish solid versus cystic structures, and to assess for the extraosseous extension of pathologic processes, but it is not essential for routine assessment of the marrow. In fact, administering gadolinium on T1-weighted sequences without fat saturation may mask pathologic processes, such as metastatic foci, which enhance and thus give a similar appearance to the adjacent, normal, fat-containing marrow, which is also bright on T1-weighted sequences. The richly vascularized red or hematopoietic marrow may enhance, particularly in children who have an abundant supply. Imaging the spine is standard in any general survey of the marrow when a diffuse marrow process is suspected or is being followed for progression.

Normal appearance of the spinal marrow

Normal marrow is composed of an intermixture of red hematopoietic marrow, yellow fatty marrow, and trabeculae in varying proportions, based on patient age and other factors. Its normal appearance on MR imaging reflects this combination. Yellow marrow, because it is composed of fatty elements, follows the signal intensity of subcutaneous fat on both T1-weighted and T2-weighted sequences. It saturates similarly to subcutaneous fat on T2-weighted sequences with fat saturation, and on STIR sequences. The resultant signal intensity is low to intermediate on T2-weighted sequences with fat saturation. The STIR sequence fully suppresses the yellow marrow signal intensity, resulting in a uniformly dark appearance. Red or hematopoietic marrow demonstrates intermediate signal intensity on T1-weighted sequences, and thus can be differentiated easily from areas of proportionally more yellow marrow. On T2-weighted sequences, the red marrow is intermediate in signal intensity, which can result in some difficulty in distinguishing red marrow from yellow marrow on this sequence. Fat saturation or STIR sequences are very useful in this case, with the red marrow demonstrating higher signal intensity than the fat-saturated yellow marrow.

The signal intensity of the red marrow is slightly higher than that of skeletal muscle, which is useful as an internal control in the evaluation of pathologic marrow changes. An important feature of normal hematopoietic or red marrow is that its signal intensity on T1-weighted sequences is just higher than that of normal muscle and the intervertebral disc because of the physiologic admixture of fatty elements in normal red marrow. When regions of marrow are as dark as, or darker than, a normal intervertebral disc or adjacent muscle on the same image, pathology is almost certainly present [4]. Because red and yellow elements coexist within normal marrow, a heterogeneous appearance of the vertebral marrow is also not uncommon. However, a focal region of a relatively high concentration of red marrow should give one pause to consider whether this may represent an area of pathology, such as an osseous metastasis. One should be able to determine the benign nature of the focal red marrow using a standard T1-weighted sequence and the internal signal characteristics, as described earlier. If not, additional sequences, such as in- and out-of-phase gradient echo sequences, may be able to provide additional information (see later discussion).

In contrast to focal red marrow collections, a focal collection of yellow marrow should not raise as much concern [4]. Degenerative disc disease can cause fatty changes in the marrow adjacent to the endplate, particularly Modic type 2 changes [2]. Additionally, it is common to see focal areas of fat within the vertebral marrow, which may be caused by alterations in vascularity. The areas of fat are especially common in the center of the vertebral bodies, in the location of the basivertebral vessels. Benign lesions, such as hemangiomas, can also appear as small foci of fat.

Pathologic considerations

Abnormalities of the spinal marrow can be classified broadly into such categories as proliferative or depletion disorders, replacement disorders, and miscellaneous disorders including such widespread entities as Paget's disease, osteopetrosis, trauma, and osteomyelitis. Many pathologic processes in the marrow have a nonspecific appearance on MR imaging, appearing low in signal intensity on T1-weighted images, and intermediate to high in signal intensity on T2-weighted images, and often demonstrate enhancement after contrast administration. However, with a careful evaluation of the location and extent of the marrow abnormalities, and an evaluation of the surrounding soft tissues,

including the intervertebral disc, a reasonable differential diagnosis can usually be made. Often, this diagnosis, combined with clinical symptoms, history, and laboratory values, can narrow the differential even further, and a specific diagnosis can be obtained. Sometimes, however, a percutaneous, or open, surgical biopsy ultimately is needed for diagnosis.

Proliferative disorders arise from the marrow elements and can be benign or malignant, encompassing disease processes ranging from polycythemia vera to leukemia. Depletion disorders involve a loss of the normal marrow elements, and can result from internal systemic processes such as aplastic anemia, or from external sources, most often radiation therapy. Replacement disorders are the result of infiltration and displacement of normal cells by cells that are not normally present within the spinal marrow. These processes may also be benign or malignant, and include benign primary bone tumors and metastatic foci. Gaucher's disease should be considered in this category; it results from the replacement of normal marrow elements by lipid-filled macrocytes, or Gaucher cells. Miscellaneous entities do not fit neatly into either of the above categories. Included here are processes that have a secondary effect on the appearance of the marrow, such as degenerative disc disease; processes that stimulate edema within the marrow, such as infectious spondylitis and acute trauma; and entities that primarily affect the bone, such as Paget's disease and osteopetrosis.

Marrow proliferative disorders

Admittedly, any categorization of the diverse entities that affect the MR appearance of the spine is artificial. However, it is useful to think in terms of broad categories so as to consider any and all possibilities, while at the same time organizing a useful differential diagnosis.

The proliferative diseases of spinal marrow result from the overgrowth of normal marrow elements, which results in a diffusely abnormal appearance of the marrow signal on MR. The signal intensity may be normal on both T1-weighted and T2-weighted sequences if the disease burden is low; or the signal intensity may be grossly abnormal in severe or advanced disease in which marrow signal is significantly lower than the T1 signal of the adjacent normal disc or muscle. Diffuse, benign processes may range from a simple, hematopoietic response to hemolytic anemia, a high-altitude environment, and even smoking, to a primary internal derangement of hematopoiesis, such as polycythemia vera or myelofibrosis.

Malignant causes that may give a diffusely abnormal appearance to spinal marrow include, but are not limited to, leukemia and Waldenstrom's macroglobulinemia (Fig. 1). One exception to the imaging appearance of malignant processes is multiple myeloma. Myeloma remains a difficult disease process to image, and correlation with laboratory results is essential. The myelomatous cells inhibit osteoblastic activity, resulting in nuclear medicine bone scans that are often negative or underestimate the disease burden. Positron emission tomography scanning has shown mixed results, and plain radiographs often take some time before the lytic lesions can be detected adequately, particularly in the spine. MR is probably the best imaging modality to detect and localize the lesions, if more to guide the biopsy than to establish a definitive diagnosis. It is also useful in following the disease progression or the response to therapy.

Although myeloma may give a diffusely abnormal pattern on MR imaging, the marrow appearance may be normal, may show well-defined focal lesions, or may have a variegated pattern [4]. The diffusely abnormal marrow pattern is seen in patients who have the most severe disease burden. These additional patterns may coexist in the same patient and represent different degrees of disease burden or response to therapy [4]. The focal lesions may have an appearance identical to metastatic

disease, with a T1-weighted signal intensity equal to, or lower than, the adjacent disc or muscle. In untreated patients, the T2-weighted signal intensity is variable, with approximately 50% of lesions showing hyperintense T2-weighted signal intensity. Also, hemorrhage into a lesion may increase its T1-weighted signal intensity. A "mini-brain" appearance has been described for focal myelomatous lesions, and it is relatively specific for this entity [4]. It results from bony struts radiating inward into the lesion from the periphery, giving the appearance of sulci and gyri in the brain. The variegated pattern appears as if cracked pepper were sprinkled onto the marrow on T1-weighted images [4]. Signal intensity on the T2-weighted images may be increased correspondingly. This pattern is also reported to be relatively specific for myeloma [4]. If patients have had MR imaging before treatment, it may be useful to assess for change in high T2 signal intensity lesions, because a successful response to therapy may show a decrease in T2-weighted signal intensity in these lesions [4]. A lack of enhancement in the lesions after gadolinium may also indicate a successful response to therapy, particularly if pretreatment contrast-enhanced MR images are available for comparison [4].

The most common form of leukemia in North America and Europe is B-cell chronic lymphocytic leukemia (CLL) (Fig. 2) [5,6]. It is characterized

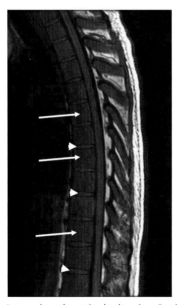

Fig. 1. Acute lymphocytic leukemia. Sagittal T1-weighted image demonstrates diffusely decreased T1 signal intensity within the vertebral bodies (*white arrows*) in the thoracic spine, which is lower than the signal intensity in normal intervertebral discs (*white arrowheads*).

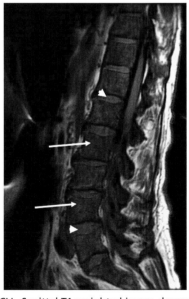

Fig. 2. CLL. Sagittal T1-weighted image demonstrates diffusely decreased T1 signal intensity within the vertebral bodies (*white arrows*) in the lumbar spine, which is lower than the signal intensity in normal thoracolumbar and lumbar intervertebral discs (*white arrowheads*).

by a monoclonal proliferation of small- or mature-appearing lymphocytes of B-cell origin [7]. These cells accumulate in the blood, spleen, lymph nodes, and marrow, and decrease normal marrow production. The diagnosis can be made by confirming an absolute lymphocytosis in the peripheral blood and in the marrow. Generally, leukemia is a diffuse process, but focal deposits have been known to occur, and can simulate metastases. MR imaging typically shows diffuse, low-signal intensity within the marrow, in comparison with muscle or intervertebral discs, on the T1-weighted sequences. The T2-weighted signal intensity typically shows higher signal than adjacent muscle because of the high water content of the leukemic cells [4].

Currently, researchers are investigating the clinical usefulness of quantitative MR imaging in evaluating the marrow, including vertebral marrow, in patients who have CLL. It is hoped that novel approaches, such as quantitative MR imaging of the marrow, may be useful in staging and in assessing response to treatment. In a study of 29 subjects who had CLL, Lecouvet and coworkers [8] found a positive synchronism between changes in lumbar marrow composition and changes in peripheral marrow composition. However, their work also demonstrated some of the limits of quantitative MR imaging in patients who have CLL, because it failed to detect any bone marrow abnormality in 41% of the subjects studied [8]. Nevertheless, quantitative MR methods continue to offer great promise in directing the clinical management of patients who have acute and chronic leukemia, and are an active area of research.

Marrow replacement disorders

Replacement disorders, simply put, are disease processes in which normal marrow elements are replaced by abnormal cells. Unlike proliferative disorders, this process typically causes focal, rather than diffuse, marrow abnormalities. The prototypical example is spinal metastases, such as from breast or prostate carcinoma. Lymphoma can be considered to be in this category also, because the lymphomatous cells are often deposited in the spinal marrow with an appearance in the spine that can be indistinguishable from metastatic disease from other causes. However, lymphoma is often low on T2-weighted and T1-weighted images.

Metastatic lesions usually are low in T1-weighted signal intensity, lower, in fact, than adjacent muscle or a normal intervertebral disc. They are often higher in signal intensity than adjacent marrow on T2-weighted sequences because of high cellular content and adjacent edema, which can be extensive. Multifocal lesions (Fig. 3) and other diagnostic

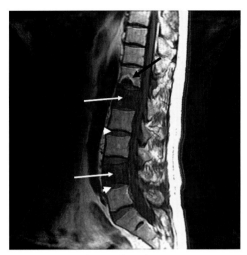

Fig. 3. Metastatic disease from breast carcinoma. Sagittal T1-weighted image demonstrates diffusely decreased T1 signal intensity within the L1 and L4 vertebral bodies (*white arrows*) in the lumbar spine, which is lower than the signal intensity in normal intervertebral discs (*white arrowheads*). An additional metastatic focus or a large Schmorl's node is present along the inferior endplate of T12 (*black arrow*).

clues, such as the involvement of a pedicle (Fig. 4) or the presence of an epidural mass, should lead one to suspect metastatic disease. Sclerotic metastatic foci, most commonly resulting from primary prostate or breast carcinoma, are often low in signal intensity on both T1- and T2-weighted sequences. MR imaging is an excellent method not only for detecting and confirming metastatic disease (from an abnormal bone scan, for example) but also for assessing response to therapy. A careful evaluation for so-called "halo signs" can be useful when evaluating metastatic disease and its response to therapy. A high T2 signal intensity rim or halo representing edema surrounding a lesion usually represents an active lesion. Conversely, a high T1 signal intensity rim or halo representing fat surrounding a lesion often indicates a treated lesion that is responding to therapy [4,9].

Primary benign and malignant bone tumors of the spine and marrow often have a nonspecific MR appearance and, when suspected, should be evaluated further with plain radiographs or CT. Their location within the vertebral body, pedicle, or posterior elements, and the level of spinal involvement, can also help in discriminating between tumors. For example, a lesion that is heterogeneous in signal intensity on T1- and T2-weighted sequences and is present in the sacrum or coccyx should raise suspicion for a chordoma, because of its characteristic location. However, on rare occasions, chordomas may arise in other locations of the spine. MR imaging is also an excellent modality

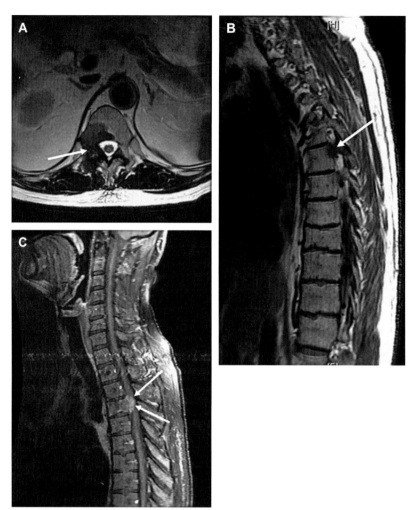

Fig. 4. Metastatic disease from colon carcinoma. (*A*) Axial FSE T2 image shows a metastatic deposit in the right pedicle (*white arrow*). (*B*) Sagittal T1-weighted image shows a low signal intensity lesion in the pedicle, consistent with a metastatic focus (*white arrow*). (*C*) Sagittal fat-saturated T1-weighted MR image of the cervicothoracic spine obtained after intravenous gadolinium administration demonstrates an enhancing metastatic lesion in the T4 vertebral body, which is protruding through the posterior aspect of the body and extending into the epidural space (*white arrows*).

for categorizing differences in tissue content between metastatic disease and primary tumors, such as an aneurismal bone cyst, which may contain characteristic fluid–fluid levels.

One benign tumor, the hemangioma, is exceedingly common, and often requires no plain film correlation or specific follow-up evaluation. Typically, hemangiomas are more common in the vertebral body than in the posterior elements, are asymptomatic, and are often multiple. Vertebral hemangiomas are round, well-defined lesions of variable size that are high in T1- and T2-weighted signal intensity. They have this appearance on T1 because of their significant fat component (Fig. 5). The appearance of higher signal intensity on the T2-weighted sequences with fat saturation

is due to the slow vascular flow in the lesions. A certain type of hemangioma has been described that contains more vessels than fat, and thus has a low signal intensity on the T1-weighted sequences and a high signal intensity on the T2-weighted sequences. Hemangiomas can also enhance diffusely with gadolinium [10]. This appearance can be identical to metastatic foci or other aggressive tumors of the bone. To complicate matters further, aggressive hemangiomas can be painful symptomatically because of fractures or collapse of the vertebral body, and can also extend into the epidural space and cause neurologic compromise [4,10]. A nuclear medicine bone scan may be effective in separating some of the less aggressive hemangiomas from metastatic disease because they typically do not

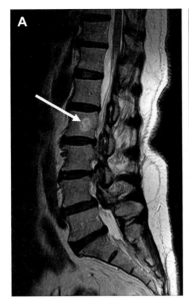 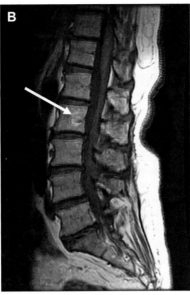

Fig. 5. Hemangioma. (*A*) Sagittal T2-weighted MR image shows a well-defined lesion in the L2 vertebral body (*white arrow*) that has increased signal intensity, compared with the surrounding marrow elements. (*B*) Sagittal T1-weighted MR image shows the same lesion to have heterogeneously high signal intensity, compared with the surrounding marrow elements (*white arrow*).

demonstrate increased uptake of Technetium 99m-methylene diphosphonate. Similar to the other characteristics of aggressive hemangiomas, these may be indistinguishable from a malignant process on the nuclear medicine bone scan because they can cause sufficient osseous disturbance to give rise to increased radiotracer uptake.

Another primary benign lesion in the spine is the bone island or enostosis. Its appearance is of diffusely low T1 and T2 signal intensity, as would be expected from the dense cortical bone that composes a bone island. Occasionally, this lesion can be confused with sclerotic metastatic disease in patients who have known or suspected metastatic disease. The absence of pain or significant activity on a bone scan can help in differentiating this from metastatic disease, as can correlation with CT or plain films that may show the typical spiculated margins that represent the blending of the enostosis with the surrounding cancellous bone.

Marrow depletion disorders

Marrow depletion is simply the absence of normal marrow elements. Its MR imaging appearance predictably shows diffuse or localized high signal intensity on T1-weighted sequences that follow fat (Fig. 6). The T2-weighted sequences correspondingly follow fat and demonstrate low signal intensity on T2-weighted sequences with fat saturation, and on STIR sequences. A common cause of marrow depletion is postradiation change in the spinal marrow, with a clear demarcation between the vertebrae within the radiation port showing diffusely high T1 signal intensity, and those outside the radiation field appearing normal. The affected regions

gradually lose marrow elements over approximately 6 weeks following therapy. In patients who have received less than 30 Gy, the hematopoietic marrow elements gradually return after a year, and the vertebral body can return to a normal appearance eventually. In patients who receive more than 50 Gy, the changes are most often permanent [4].

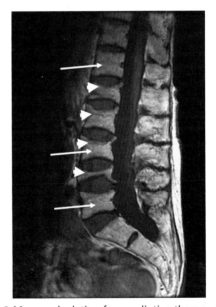

Fig. 6. Marrow depletion from radiation therapy. Sagittal T1-weighted MR image shows diffusely high T1 signal intensity throughout the thoracolumbar spine (*white arrows*). Multiple compression fractures are also present (*white arrowheads*), as may be seen commonly in patients after radiation therapy. This portion of the spine was in a radiation port.

The appearance of the spinal marrow of aplastic anemia and postchemotherapy patients is identical to that of radiation change; however, all of the vertebral bodies are involved. It is important to determine how much chemotherapy the patient has received because the marrow may appear surprisingly normal after some regimens. It is also important to ascertain whether the patient has received medication to stimulate the marrow, such as colony-stimulating factors. The marrow, on stimulation, may demonstrate focal regions or islands of actively regenerating hematopoietic marrow surrounded by fat, which may be mistaken for disease recurrence, particularly metastatic foci.

Miscellaneous marrow abnormalities

Degenerative disc disease

Degenerative disc disease can cause changes in the MR imaging appearance of the adjacent bone marrow and endplates in the spine [11]. Three different types of change were described initially by Modic, affecting 22% to 50% of discs in subjects who had degenerative disc disease [2,11].

Modic type I lesions demonstrate hypointense marrow and endplates on T1-weighted sequences, and hyperintense marrow and endplates on T2-weighted sequences, and are thought to represent an active degenerative process. Toyone and coworkers [12] found an association between Modic type I changes and low back pain, and Mitra and coworkers [13] found a trend of symptom improvement and the evolution of type I to type II changes. Modic type II lesions are hyperintense on both T1-weighted and T2-weighted sequences, and are thought to represent fatty degeneration of the marrow, a more chronic and stable process [2]. They are often thought to progress from type I changes. Modic type III changes are hypointense on both T1-weighted and T2-weighted sequences, and are thought to correlate with subchondral sclerosis [2]. Kuisma and coworkers [14] studied 60 nonoperative sciatica patients with baseline and 3-year follow-up MR imaging to assess the prevalence and natural course of Modic changes over a 3-year follow-up period. A prevalence of 23% was detected, similar to previous studies, with 79% of changes occurring at the L4–L5 and the L5–S1 levels. These changes had a positive correlation with patient age. They also found that 14% of the discs with baseline Modic changes displayed a different type at follow-up, and that those that did not change type increased in size. The incidence of new Modic changes at 3-year follow-up was 6%. Their study also demonstrated Modic type II changes may convert to another type, suggesting

a superimposed change, such as superimposed or continued degeneration [14].

Schmorl's nodes represent vertical disc prolapses through areas of weakness in the vertebral body endplate. They may be caused by any disorder that weakens the endplate or the subchondral bone, and they may be associated with trauma. They are observed often on MR imaging evaluation of the spine [15], and usually are clearly recognized by the contour defect and the disc protruding into the endplate. Grive and coworkers [15] described two cases of acute Schmorl's nodes in which MR showed a decreased vertebral T1 signal and a slightly increased T2 signal, which are typical with inflammatory response. Schmorl's nodes also typically demonstrate a rim of enhancement after contrast administration. Unfortunately, these signal characteristics are indistinguishable from a host of infectious and inflammatory processes. A careful search for an endplate defect or an intranuclear cleft bending of the disc may help diagnose this entity correctly.

Spinal infections

Infectious spondylitis and spondylodiscitis comprise the next broad category of pathologic processes that affect the MR imaging appearance of the marrow. Pyogenic spondylodiscitis represents approximately 2% to 4% of all cases of osteomyelitis [16–20]. The most common mechanism of infection is through an arterial hematogenous spread from distant septic foci, although venous spread through Batson's perivertebral plexus, contiguous spread from adjacent soft tissues, and direct inoculation following surgery or percutaneous diagnostic or therapeutic procedures have all been described. In children, the vascular supply within the immature intervertebral disc and the adjacent cartilaginous vertebral body endplates is abundant. These vascular channels of the immature disc and capillary tufts in the endplates are thought to predispose the child to discitis. Blood supply to the intervertebral disc usually disappears by age 20. In adults, the primary site of infection becomes the vertebral body, with secondary discitis due to osteomyelitis or from a contiguous paravertebral abscess. The arterial anatomy of the vertebral body explains the pathogenesis of vertebral osteomyelitis and discitis. The metaphysis, particularly the anterior–lateral portion, is susceptible to osteomyelitis because of the greater number of arteries within it, compared with the equator or central portion of the vertebral body. It is believed that septic microemboli lodge in the metaphyseal arteries [21].

Vertebral osteomyelitis is distributed bimodally, with a prominent peak in adults older than 50 and a smaller peak in the second decade [16]. The lumbar spine is the most common area of involvement, although any area can be affected. The causative organism varies with age, geographic location, and underlying medical conditions; however, gram-positive and gram-negative pyogenic bacteria are the most frequent causative organisms in the developed world. *Staphlococcus aureus* was found to be the dominant organism in many series [16,22]. Commonly, infections of the spine demonstrate low T1 signal intensity, high T2 signal intensity, and enhancement within the affected marrow after gadolinium administration. These marrow abnormalities and enhancement patterns, however, can be nonspecific (Fig. 7). Therefore, diagnosing spondylitis is not always easy, particularly when the infection is in its early phase, is located in an atypical location, or occurs in regions of pre-existing degenerative disc disease, or when the tumor is located in the vertebral body immediately adjacent to the disc (myeloma-chordoma) [23]. Most of the time, however, disease recognition based on MR imaging patterns can help differentiate infectious causes of marrow abnormalities from various neoplastic, inflammatory, degenerative, systemic, metabolic, and traumatic causes.

Evaluation patterns should include a thorough assessment of the intervertebral discs and vertebral body endplates. Disc findings of pyogenic spondylodiscitis include decreased disc height,

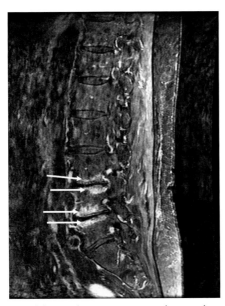

Fig. 7. Endplate enhancement secondary to degenerative disc disease. Sagittal T1-weighted MR image with fat saturation obtained after intravenous gadolinium administration demonstrates bandlike enhancement of the vertebral endplates (*white arrows*) adjacent to the L3–L4 and the L4–L5 intervertebral discs, which are degenerated.

disc hypointensity on T1-weighted images, disc hyperintensity on T2-weighted images, and diffuse disc enhancement. Vertebral bodies typically show endplate erosion and signal alterations (ie, decreased T1 signal and increased T2 signal) immediately adjacent to the affected disc. Ledermann and coworkers [24] reviewed contrast-enhanced MR images of 46 consecutive patients with culture or histologic examination results positive for spondylodiscitis, and concluded that imaging criteria with good-to-excellent sensitivity for spinal infection should include: (1) evidence of either a paraspinal or epidural inflammatory tissue, (2) contrast enhancement of the disc, (3) fluid signal intensity on T2-weighted images, and, finally, (4) erosion or destruction of the vertebral endplates on T1-weighted images (Fig. 8) [24]. Unfortunately, they also showed that atypical manifestations of spinal infection may not result in the classic imaging patterns. Rarely, involvement may be limited to one vertebral body, a vertebral body and adjacent disc, or the epidural space, exclusively. Furthermore, in hematogenous spread, infections frequently involve several spinal levels. They concluded that criteria with limited clinical use and a low sensitivity included hypointensity of the disc on T1-weighted images and decreased intervertebral disc height. Also, effacement of the internuclear cleft on T2-weighted images is rarely applicable in the thoracic and cervical spine [24].

Tuberculosis (TB) is caused by *Mycobacterium tuberculosis*. It remains a major public heath hazard in the developing world, and its incidence has been increasing in the developed world since the 1990s. The reasons for the increased incidence are multifactorial, but they are related in large part to immunosuppression, most notably in patients infected with human immunodeficiency virus, and to immigration from countries where TB is endemic [25].

Spinal TB can cause serious morbidity resulting from paraplegia, and sometimes even quadriplegia, which occurs in approximately 10% of cases [26,27]. Tuberculous infections of the spine (Pott's disease) may also result in a significant kyphotic deformity, even without neurologic impairment. Spinal TB accounts for more than 50% of musculoskeletal TB [28]. It is therefore imperative to consider this diagnosis in all cases of suspected infectious spondylitis of the spine, to enable timely, antimicrobial, and even sometimes surgical, treatment, in the hope of preventing serious spinal deformity and neurologic morbidity.

Spinal TB is most often a secondary infection, caused by hematogenous spread from a pulmonary or genitourinary source. The incidence of extrapulmonary tuberculous infection increases in the

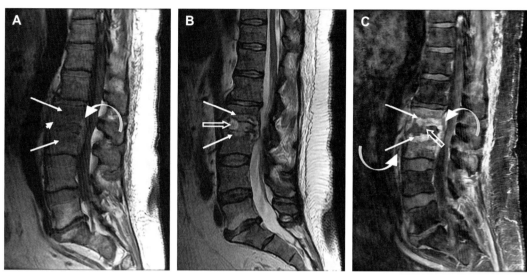

Fig. 8. Pyogenic spondylodiscitis. (*A*) Sagittal T1-weighted image shows endplate destruction (*white arrowhead*) and low signal intensity in the L2 and L3 vertebral bodies (*white arrows*). An epidural phlegmon or abscess is also present (*curved white arrow*). (*B*) Sagittal T2-weighted MR image shows corresponding high T2 signal intensity in the intervertebral disc (*open white arrow*) and the vertebral bodies (*white arrows*) at the L2–L3 level. (*C*) Sagittal fat-saturated T1-weighted MR image obtained after intravenous gadolinium administration shows enhancement in the disc space (*open white arrow*), and vertebral bodies (*white arrows*) at the L2–L3 level, and also demonstrates inflammatory phlegmon anterior and posterior to the vertebral bodies (*curved white arrows*).

elderly and the immunocompromised. The most frequent site of spinal involvement is at the thoracolumbar junction, usually in the lower thoracic spine. However, infection limited to the cervical spine, the lumbar spine, and even the cranioverte-bral junction, has been reported [29]. The infection commonly begins in the anterior aspect of the vertebral body adjacent to the intervertebral disc, then spreads to adjacent discs under the anterior longitudinal ligament. This process often results in characteristic noncontiguous, or skip, lesions, involving multiple vertebral bodies. Despite extensive bony involvement and destruction, the disc spaces are relatively preserved, a finding that is virtually pathognomonic for spinal TB [25]. Disc involvement is thought to be delayed because *Mycobacterium TB* lacks specific cartilage proteolytic enzymes [23]. Isolated involvement of the posterior elements of the spine has been described [30].

The marrow response to infection is nonspecific, and therefore its characteristic imaging appearance on MR imaging, including low T1-weighted signal intensity, high T2-weighted signal intensity, and enhancement following gadolinium administration, is present in both tuberculous and pyogenic infections. However, Jung and coworkers [28] found that MR imaging was accurate for differentiating tuberculous spondylitis from pyogenic spondylitis using a careful evaluation of the pattern of marrow involvement and the appearance of the surrounding soft tissue. They determined that the presence of a well-defined, paraspinal, abnormal signal, a thin and smooth abscess wall, subligamen-tous spread to three or more vertebral levels, multiple or entire vertebral involvement, and thoracic spine involvement were more suggestive of tuberculous spondylitis than pyogenic spondylitis (Fig. 9) [28]. The reviewer identified tuberculous spondylitis with a sensitivity, specificity, and accuracy of 100 %, 80%, and 90%, respectively [28]. Given the differences in the choice and length of antimicrobial therapy and the potential need for operative treatment, a percutaneous or open biopsy is often needed for confirmation. The key role of the radiologist lies in suspecting and suggesting the diagnosis, so that the appropriate laboratory tests, ancillary imaging, and initial patient therapeutic and management considerations can be made

Brucellosis is a zoonosis with a worldwide distribution. It is unusual in developed countries, but is a relatively common cause of vertebral osteomyelitis in some areas of the world, such as Latin America, the Middle East, and the Mediterranean, where *Brucella melitenses* is endemic [31]. Osteoarticular disease is the most common complication of brucellosis and has been described in 10% to 85% of patients [31–33]. Spondylodiscitis is a common manifestation of osteoarticular involvement in adults and, like tuberculous spondylodiscitis, can result in spinal deformities and neurologic deficits.

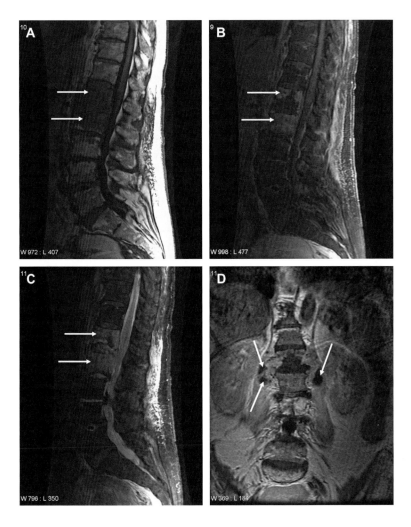

Fig. 9. Tuberculous spondylitis (*A*) Sagittal T1-weighted MR image shows abnormally low T1 signal intensity in the L1 and L2 vertebral bodies (*white arrows*). (*B*) Sagittal T1-weighted MR image with fat saturation obtained after intravenous administration of gadolinium shows abnormal enhancement in the L1 and L2 vertebral bodies (*white arrows*). (*C*) Sagittal T2-weighted MR image with fat saturation shows abnormally high signal intensity in the L1 and L2 vertebral bodies (*white arrows*). (*D*) Coronal T1-weighted MR image obtained after intravenous administration of gadolinium shows non-enhancing bilateral psoas muscle abscesses (*white arrows*) located just lateral to the L1-2 intervertebral disc.

Brucellar spondylodiscitis may have an acute or chronic course, and may present with mild and nonspecific clinical symptoms. Timely diagnosis is also hindered by the frequently long latent period between the onset of symptoms and the appearance of radiologic findings (2–8 weeks) [31]. The MR imaging appearances of both brucellar spondylitis and tuberculous spondylitis can demonstrate extensive paraspinal inflammation and abscesses; however, the size of the paraspinal mass may be larger in TB than in brucellosis. Harman and coworkers [31] evaluated 25 subjects who had brucellar spondylitis and found slight differences in the MR imaging appearance in subjects who had acute, versus chronic, brucellar spondylitis. They found that in subjects who had acute vertebral brucellar infection (7 to 20 days after clinical presentation), the intervertebral discs and adjacent vertebral bodies showed T1 hypointense and T2 hyperintense signal, similar to pyogenic infection. As infection became chronic (3 to 6 weeks after the clinical onset), disc and endplate signal could vary considerably;

however, the vertebral bodies were all inhomogeneous in appearance. Thus, brucellar spondylitis can give imaging appearances similar to pyogenic spondylodiscitis, with characteristic disc and adjacent vertebral body involvement, and also tuberculous spondylodiscitis, with significant paraspinal involvement, and can even have a varied MR imaging appearance, based on its chronicity.

Inflammatory conditions

Ankylosing spondylitis is a chronic inflammatory disease that affects the sacroiliac joints and the spine. MR imaging has represented a major advance in the early diagnosis of ankylosing spondylitis, particularly with the advent of fat-suppressed T2-weighted sequences that allow early detection of bone marrow edema and inflammation in the sacroiliac joints and spine. MR imaging is able to detect inflammation earlier than plain film radiography, and thus has important diagnostic and therapeutic benefits, because causes of back pain can vary widely.

Osteitis in ankylosing spondylitis appears as low signal intensity regions on T1-weighted images and correspondingly as high signal intensity regions on T2-weighted sequences, consistent with inflammation; the high signal intensity regions are particularly apparent when the T2-weighted fat saturation technique is used. These areas also enhance following gadolinium administration. The MR imaging findings can be observed with or without corresponding abnormalities on plain films. Also, inflammatory changes may be confined to the corners of vertebral bodies or may be distributed more widely [34]. Plain film findings in the spine in ankylosing spondylitis are well-described, and include focal erosions along the anterior margin of the discovertebral junction at the superior and inferior aspects of the vertebral bodies, which are referred to as Romulus lesions [35]. These erosions produce an appearance of squared-off vertebrae. Later, in the healing phase, reactive sclerosis occurs, giving the "shiny corner" appearance [36]. On MR imaging, regions of inflammation may be identified as low T1, high T2 signal intensity foci that enhance with gadolinium, representing active inflammation. This appearance of noninfectious osteitis by MR imaging can appear long before the frank osseous erosions and subsequent repair can be identified on radiographs.

Kurugoglu and coworkers [34] studied five patients who had low back pain, with contrast enhanced MR imaging. All had normal plain film evaluation of the spine and sacroiliac joints. MR imaging showed both vertebral body and endplate involvement with low T1 and high T2 signal, and all lesions enhanced after gadolinium. Two patients showed disease in both the thoracic and lumbar regions, whereas the remaining three showed disease confined to the lumbar spine. In the thoracolumbar spine, changes were contiguous, with widespread signal alteration affecting vertebral bodies, endplates, and pedicles. In comparison, disease limited to the lumbar spine showed confinement of pathologic signal to the corners of vertebral bodies. The spinal canal and the paravertebral areas had no accompanying soft tissue masses, and the intervertebral disc spaces and disc signal intensities were normal. Subsequent work-up confirmed a diagnosis of ankylosing spondylitis. They concluded that patients who have early and undiagnosed ankylosing spondylitis, especially adolescents who do not have a typical history or who have plain radiographic findings, may present with the above described MR findings [34].

Although these MR imaging findings are somewhat nonspecific and may be present in many benign or aggressive disease processes, an awareness of the MR appearance of osteitis will help raise the suspicion of ankylosing spondylitis. Then, with further radiographic evaluation of the signal intensity joints, and clinical and serologic evaluation with a search for the HLA-B27 antigen, the appropriate diagnosis can be made.

Special considerations

Red marrow reconversion–sickle cell anemia

The bone marrow is producing red blood cells constantly, which have an average life span of approximately 120 days. In patients who have sickle cell anemia, affected red blood cells instead have a life span of approximately 10 to 20 days, which forces the marrow to replace red blood cells continually as a result of a severe, chronic anemia. Skeletal complications of this disease have been studied extensively; the degree of spinal involvement depends on the duration and severity of the disease and is more common during and after the second decade [37].

The spinal vertebral bodies are affected by erythroid hyperplasia, which destroys the normal trabeculae. The normal trabeculae is then replaced by connective tissue, which results in vertebral body weakness and collapse, further complicated by vaso-occlusion, infarction, and ischemia. Red marrow reconversion, which occurs in sickle cell anemia (and in other diseases such as thalassemia), begins in the axial skeleton and then progresses to involve the appendicular skeleton. Advanced red marrow reconversion results in significant replacement of the yellow marrow by hematopoietic elements and therefore a rather homogeneous low T1 signal intensity in the vertebral bodies. This low T1 signal may, in fact, be lower than in an adjacent intervertebral disc or muscle. Lesser degrees of red marrow reconversion have been reported to occur in obese women [4] and in smokers, but give the marrow a more heterogeneous appearance on T1. In sickle cell anemia, the appearance of the thoracic and lumbar vertebrae on MR imaging often shows diffusely low T1-signal intensity as a result of marrow hyperplasia, with a signal intensity lower than the intervertebral discs (Fig. 10). In addition, hemosiderin deposition from the chronic destruction of red blood cells, which occurs in sickle cell anemia and other blood dyscrasias such as thalassemia, can result further in uniformly low signal intensity on T1-weighted, T2-weighted, and gradient echo sequences. The T2-signal intensity in sickle cell anemia can vary from areas of hypointensity to hyperintensity, depending on the presence of hemosiderin deposition, ischemia, infarction, and recent collapse.

The shapes of the vertebral bodies are distinct and often demonstrate patterns of vertebral ischemia collectively called "Reynolds' vertebrae," or so-called "fish-" or "H-shaped vertebrae," previously

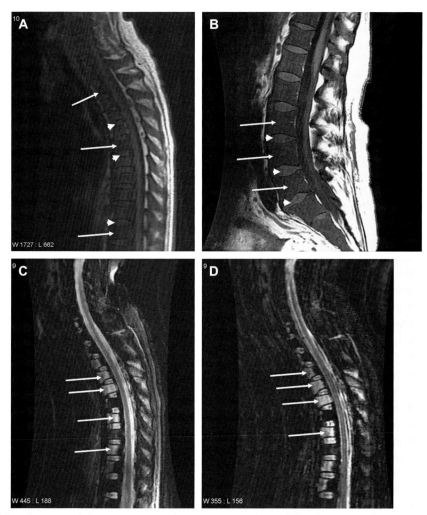

Fig. 10. Sickle cell anemia. (*A*) Sagittal T1-weighted MR image shows diffusely low signal intensity in the vertebral bodies (*white arrows*), which is lower than the signal in the corresponding intervertebral discs (*white arrowheads*). (*B*) Sagittal T1-weighted MR image in another patient also shows diffusely low signal intensity in the vertebral bodies (*white arrows*), which is lower than the signal in the corresponding intervertebral discs (*white arrowheads*). (*C*) Sagittal FSE T2-weighted MR image with fat saturation, and (*D*) sagittal STIR sequences show heterogeneous areas of increased signal intensity (*white arrows*), which likely represent areas of infarction in this patient who has acute thoracic pain.

described on plain radiographs (Fig. 11) [38]. Recently, Marlow and coworkers [39] described a phenomenon called "tower vertebrae," which are thought to represent a compensatory increase in the vertical height of thoracic vertebrae in response to childhood infarction and subsequent hypoplasia of adjacent vertebrae.

Vertebral osteomyelitis may further complicate sickle cell anemia, and needs to be considered in any patient who has sickle cell disease and is presenting with back pain, because timely diagnosis and treatment are essential to avoid significant morbidity. Sadat-Ali and coworkers [37] studied 34 patients between the ages of 4 and 28 who sought treatment for complications of sickle cell disease.

They found infectious spondylitis in eight patients (24%), which was caused by Staphlococcus aureus, Salmonella enteriditis, and anaerobic streptococci species. In the series by Sadat-Ali and colleagues [37], Salmonella enteriditis was the causative organism in all of the children with infectious spondylitis, but Staphlococcus aureus and streptococci were the causative agent in the adults. Ultimately, surgical or percutaneous biopsy confirmation may be needed to determine the causative organism and to tailor antimicrobial therapy appropriately.

Sarcoidosis
Sarcoidosis is a multisystem disorder characterized by the presence of noncaseating granulomas in

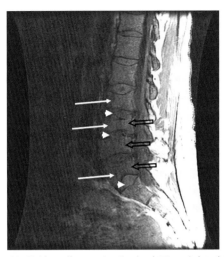

Fig. 11. Sickle cell anemia. Sagittal T1-weighted MR image of the lumbar spine demonstrates diffusely low signal intensity in the vertebral bodies (*white arrows*), which is as low as, or lower than, the signal intensity in the corresponding intervertebral discs (*white arrowheads*). Multiple biconcave vertebral bodies are present (*open black arrows*), which are the MR imaging equivalent of fish vertebrae, that occurred secondary to infarction and collapse. This process is typical of that for sickle cell anemia.

the lungs, lymph nodes, skin, visceral organs, neurologic system, and musculoskeletal system. Vertebral sarcoid described on MR imaging has been reported rarely in the literature. The MR imaging findings have been similar to CT findings, which have shown purely lytic-to-sclerotic lesions, but the MR findings are more variable [40]. Sarcoidosis should be considered in any patient who has sarcoidosis and is presenting with low back pain. The generally reported MR imaging features are low T1 signal, and high T2 signal intensity lesions that enhance following gadolinium. Unfortunately, these findings are similar to osseous metastatic lesions.

Three types of enhancement patterns have been described in sarcoid, including dense homogeneous enhancement [41], faint homogeneous enhancement [42], and peripheral inhomogeneous enhancement [43–45]. Lisle and coworkers [46] reported a case of biopsy-confirmed vertebral sarcoidosis that demonstrated low T1 signal intensity lesions that intensely and homogeneously enhanced postgadolinium. The lesions, however, were low in T2-weighted signal intensity and high on STIR sequences. This finding had not been reported previously. Furthermore, they stated that some of the larger lesions had low signal intensity centers on STIR, producing a target-like appearance. Le Breton and coworkers [42] previously had reported an absence of abnormal findings on

a bone scan. A nuclear medicine bone scan on this patient showed a mild heterogeneous increase in activity throughout the thoracic and the lumbar spine, and most of the lesions present on the MR imaging showed no sclerotic or destructive foci on CT. This example nicely illustrates the variable imaging appearance of vertebral sarcoidosis. Despite the variability in appearance, MR imaging is probably the most sensitive imaging modality for detecting vertebral sarcoidosis, and it is currently an excellent way to identify a suitable location for biopsy confirmation.

Crystalline arthropathies

Tophaceous gout rarely affects the spine, but when it does occur it can result in pain, fever, and elevated C-reactive protein, often mimicking infection [47]. Patients usually have an underlying history of polyarticular tophaceous gout within the appendicular skeleton, and the lumbar and cervical spine are involved most commonly [48]. The gouty tophi result in homogeneous, hypointense masses on both T1- and T2-weighted sequences, continuous with the facet joints and strongly enhancing [48–50]. Crystal deposition is believed to start in the facet joint and spread through the ligamentum flavum [49].

Calcium pyrophosphate deposition disease crystal deposition can affect the spine and mimic infection as well. It can result in a neuropathic appearance with destruction, vertebral collapse, and erosions after crystal deposition in the intervertebral discs, joint capsules, synovium, articular cartilage, and ligaments [51]. MR imaging often shows changes in the disc, with adjacent endplate erosive changes and marrow edema [52].

Storage diseases

Gaucher's disease is the most common lysosomal storage disorder. It is inherited as an autosomal recessive trait and involves an inborn error of glycosphingolipid metabolism. It is caused by a defect in glucocerebrosidase activity, which results in the accumulation of glucocerebrosides within the lysosomes of macrophages, called Gaucher cells. This process results in a multisystem disease that includes replacement of normal bone marrow with the lipid-laden macrophages (Gaucher cells). Patients often suffer anemia, coagulation abnormalities, hepatosplenomegaly, and structural skeletal changes [53].

Skeletal involvement varies widely, but affects approximately 75% to 80 % of patients in some form. It can range from mild osteopenia to medullary expansion and remodeling, to osteonecrosis, pathologic fractures, and vertebral body collapse [54]. Vertebral body collapse may result in neurologic compromise. Symptoms of musculoskeletal involvement range from a chronic dull ache to an acute severe episode of pain called a bone crisis [55]. The latter symptom usually is attributed to osteonecrosis, but pathologic fractures or osteomyelitis may also be responsible [56,57].

The severity of skeletal changes depends on the degree of infiltration of the marrow by the Gaucher cells [54], and MR imaging is very sensitive to the detection of this (Fig. 12). The MR imaging findings may be correlated with the patient's symptoms [54]. Based on the distribution of the abnormal marrow and the signal intensity of the marrow abnormalities, clinical behavior can be deduced [54]. For example, when the altered marrow signal intensity is low on both T1- and T2-weighted images, the normal marrow is characterized by extensive fibrosis; patients with this marrow appearance have no clinical disease [54]. However, if the abnormal marrow is low in signal intensity on T1-weighted sequences, but is of high signal intensity on T2-weighted images, this indicates active disease. Patients with this marrow appearance usually have symptoms of pain [54]. MR imaging is also useful in evaluating patients who have Gaucher's disease for bone infarction and ischemic necrosis [54], and can also identify acute to subacute compression fractures in the spine.

A careful examination of the marrow in patients who have known Gaucher's disease should be performed to assess for infectious spondylitis, because patients have an increased incidence of osteomyelitis and lymphoproliferative disorders, such as CLL, multiple myeloma, lymphoma, Hodgkin's and non-Hodgkin's lymphoma [58,59]. Shiran and coworkers [59] demonstrated a 14.7 fold increase in hematologic malignancies and a 3.6 fold increase in other types of malignancy in 48 patients who had Gaucher's disease, versus control subjects [53,59].

The bone marrow fat content is depressed in patients who have Gaucher's disease because of the displacement of marrow adipocytes by Gaucher cells. The amount of marrow fat displaced by Gaucher cells could be used as a disease marker, and quantitative CT has been used to measure this process [60]. Rosenthal and coworkers [60] described the usefulness of MR imaging in evaluating patients who have known Gaucher's disease through providing quantitative measurements of each vertebral fat fraction. This measurement correlated favorably with markers of disease severity, such as the clinical history of skeletal complications, and the hematocrit and acid phosphatase activity. Vertebral body fat fraction, as calculated by MR imaging, combined with various other techniques, can aid in following disease progression and help assess skeletal response to enzyme replacement therapy [60]. Finally, a close inspection of the paravertebral tissues should be made in patients who have Gaucher's disease. Poll and coworkers [53] reported a case of a 76-year-old woman with long-standing Gaucher's disease with cortical destruction in the thoracic vertebrae with contiguous paravertebral masses, which were consistent with extraosseous extension skeletal disease.

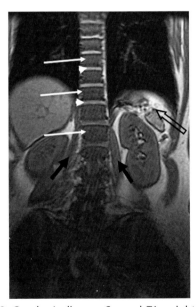

Fig. 12. Gaucher's disease. Coronal T1-weighted MR image shows diffusely low signal intensity in the vertebral bodies of the thoracolumbar spine (*white arrows*), which are lower in signal intensity than the adjacent muscles (*black arrows*) and the intervertebral discs (*white arrowheads*). The patient has had a prior partial splenectomy (*open black arrow*).

Abnormalities of the bone

Abnormalities of the cortical bone and trabeculae can affect the normal appearance of the vertebrae. Two examples are Paget's disease and osteopetrosis. Paget's disease can have a variable appearance, including areas of normal fatty marrow that demonstrate high T1 signal intensity intermixed with regions of low T1 signal intensity, which represent areas of thickened trabeculae, uncalcified osteoid, fibrovascular connective tissue, and even dilated vascular channels. The vertebral body or bodies affected may appear enlarged. Any suspicion of Paget's disease should prompt the clinician to obtain conventional radiographs, CT, or nuclear medicine correlation. Rarely, sarcomatous degeneration may occur, or metastatic foci may localize to pagetoid bone because of its relative hypervascularity, appearing as other primary bone tumors or metastatic foci would in bone, with low T1 signal and high T2 signal intensity lesions that often enhance.

In osteopetrosis, osteoclastic activity is decreased. Depending on the severity of the disease, the normal marrow space is decreased or nearly obliterated and the classic bone-in-bone appearance on plain radiographs may be seen as areas of low T1 signal intensity in the otherwise normal high T1 signal intense area within the marrow. In both Paget's disease and osteopetrosis, the bone is weaker than normal bone, and a search for pathologic fractures in addition to sarcomatous degeneration in cases of Paget's disease must be made in patients complaining of localized pain.

Severe systemic illness

It is important to mention a process called serous atrophy or gelatinous transformation of the marrow in patients suffering from severe cachexia from eating disorders or severe systemic illnesses such as HIV/AIDS. The marrow itself can become necrotic and fluid-filled [61], beginning peripherally but eventually affecting the axial skeleton. In advanced cases, the marrow follows pure fluid signal intensity on all pulse sequences [4].

Considerations in vertebral body collapse

Vertebral body collapse poses a frequent diagnostic dilemma for the radiologist and the clinician. Evaluation of the underlying cause of acute compression fractures secondary to trauma in a previously normal individual is usually straightforward; however, assessing compression fractures that have occurred with relatively little trauma can be problematic.

The vertebral body collapse may be secondary to underlying osteoporosis, which is the most frequent cause (Fig. 13). It is estimated that in the United States, 25% of postmenopausal women have a vertebral compression fracture (VCF), and this prevalence increases steadily with age [62,63].

To optimize diagnostic accuracy, an evaluation of the marrow signal characteristics, enhancement pattern, distribution of the marrow abnormalities on other areas of the spine, the vertebral body morphology, and involvement of the intervertebral disc and paraspinal soft tissue must be made. The various signs of benignity and malignancy in cases of vertebral body collapse are summarized by Tehranzadeh and Tao [63]. Signs favoring benignity in vertebral collapse include the presence of normal fatty marrow in the vertebral body, the absence of multifocal involvement or of pedicle involvement, the presence of a fracture line, the absence of a convex cortical contour or extraosseous mass, the presence of intervertebral fluid or air, and fragmentation with or without a posteriorly angulated fragment. Signs favoring malignancy conversely include the absence of normal fatty marrow, multifocal and pedicle involvement, the absence of a fracture line, intervertebral air or fluid, the absence of fragmentation or a posterior angulated fragment, the presence of a convex cortical contour, and an extraosseous soft tissue mass [63].

The investigators further summarize highly predictive findings in infectious causes of vertebral collapse, which include intense enhancement of the intervertebral disc, intense enhancement of paraspinal and or epidural extension, and intense

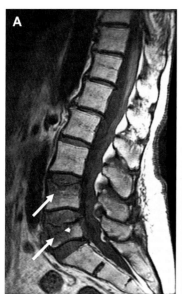 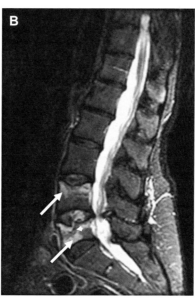

Fig. 13. Osteoporotic compression fracture. (*A*) Sagittal T1 and (*B*) sagittal T2 with fat saturation show acute-to-subacute compression fractures of the L4 and L5 vertebral bodies (*white arrows*). Only the superior portion of the L4 vertebral body and the superior and anterior portions of the L5 vertebral body demonstrate abnormal signal intensity, and a small fracture line is present in the L5 vertebral body (*white arrowhead*). A subsequent follow-up MR image (not shown) demonstrated a return of the normal T1 and T2 signal intensity in these regions.

enhancement of endplate and adjacent marrow (Fig. 14). They characterize a hyperintense disc on T2-weighted images and destruction of the endplate in T1-weighted images as fairly predictive characteristics in infectious collapse [63]. Diffusion-weighted images have been noted to demonstrate hyperintensity in both infectious and malignant causes of collapse, and so it not useful in differentiating between these two causes at this point. However, diffusion-weighted sequences have shown hypointensity in osteoporotic collapse, and so may be useful in differentiating between benign osteoporotic vertebral body collapse and infectious or malignant collapse.

Postoperative and posttherapeutic spine

Percutaneous vertebroplasty

Percutaneous vertebroplasty (PV) for treatment of VCFs was first performed in North America in 1993 and first reported in 1997 [64]. Since that time, vertebroplasty has become a well-accepted technique for the treatment of VCFs. Currently, PV is an accepted treatment for both osteoporotic and neoplastic symptomatic compression fractures. This section focuses primarily on treatment of osteoporotic VCFs.

Accurate localization of back pain to a compressed vertebral body can be difficult because numerous other processes may result in back pain, even when the pain can be localized to a particular vertebral level. Frequent mimickers include herniated discs, facet joint arthropathy, and spinal stenosis. The success of PV may hinge on appropriate patient selection, which can be difficult, particularly when the age of the compression fracture is unknown. Although some researchers have shown that chronic VCFs may benefit from PV [65,66], others have described poor treatment results when fractures have existed for more than 12 months [64]. A recent study by Tanigawa and coworkers [67] has suggested that pain relief provided by PV is proportional to the extent of bone marrow edema seen on preprocedural MR imaging.

MR imaging for pretreatment evaluation is often preferred to other diagnostic studies, such as plain film or bone scan [68,69]. Although plain films can assess the degree of fracture accurately, the chronicity cannot be assessed with comparison films. Bone scans are sensitive for detection of VCF, but anatomic information is limited, and they can show uptake long after substantial healing has occurred [69]. Many interventionalists rely on MR imaging to assist in selecting patients who have acute-to-subacute fractures (less than 45 days old) and no other causes of pain. Approximately 1 to 3 months after compression, most VCFs will heal and should return to normal signal intensity [70], although others have found that marrow edema can persist up to 48 months after the event [71]. Anatomic depiction with MR imaging allows exclusion of other disease processes, and evaluation of bone marrow edema, particularly in the setting of multiple adjacent compression fractures or prolonged pain after an inciting event.

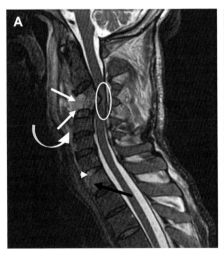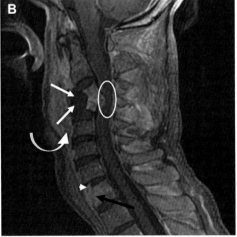

Fig. 14. Infectious vertebral body collapse. (*A*) Sagittal T2-weighted MR image with fat saturation and (*B*) sagittal fat-saturated T1-weighted MR image obtained after intravenous injection of gadolinium show collapse of the C3 vertebral body (*white arrows*) as a result of osteomyelitis and intraosseous abscess, which results in a narrowing of the spinal canal (*area within white circle*) and may lead to severe neurologic sequelae. Note the phlegmonous tissue in the prevertebral space (*curved white arrow*). The C7 vertebral body and the C6–7 intervertebral disc (*white arrowhead*) also demonstrate findings consistent with spondylodiscitis.

After PV, bone marrow signal intensity may not return to normal. Marrow edema may persist for 6 months or longer. In a study by Dansie and coworkers [72], although most patients demonstrated decreasing amounts of bone marrow edema, 22% had moderate-to-severe edema even after 6 months, and 19% developed edema in previously normal marrow. Another study by Voormolen and coworkers [71] demonstrated that 65% of patients will have edema 3 months postvertebroplasty, with one third still demonstrating edema at 1 year posttreatment, unrelated to pain. Therefore, persistent marrow edema does not appear to be a sign of ongoing symptoms in patients after PV.

Some investigators have found a significant increase in new VCFs after PV [73,74], occurring immediately adjacent to previously treated levels (Fig. 15) [75]. It has been suggested that this may be secondary to cement leakage into the disc during PV or to the increased stiffness of the vertebral body treated with polymethyl methacrylate [76].

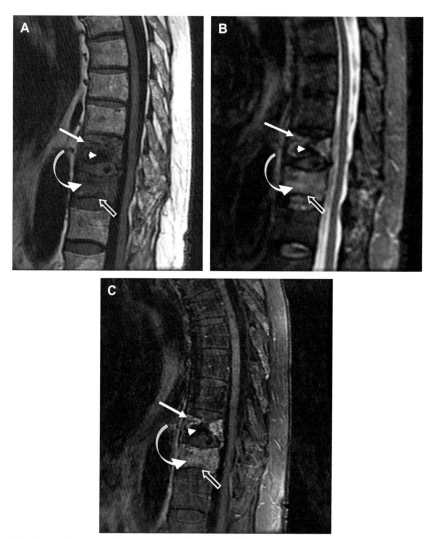

Fig. 15. Post-PV with adjacent level compression fracture. (*A*) Sagittal T1-weighted MR image, (*B*) sagittal T2-weighted image with fat saturation, and (*C*) sagittal STIR MR image demonstrate a low signal intensity region (*white arrowheads*) within a partially compressed T10 vertebral body, which represents the polymethyl methacrylate that was injected at the time of the vertebroplasty. Edema is also present within the remainder of the T10 vertebral body that is characterized by regions of decreased signal on the T1-weighted image and regions of increased signal on the fluid-sensitive sequences (*white arrows*). Note the edema (*curved white arrows*) and the slight compression deformity (*open white arrows*) of the subjacent T11 vertebral body, which represents an acute adjacent-level compression fracture adjacent to a location of recent vertebroplasty. This patient presented with acute pain approximately 6 months after a T10 vertebroplasty.

Postoperative spondylodiscitis

Postoperative spondylodiscitis is a known complication of lumbar disc surgery, occurring in approximately 0.1% to 3% of patients (Fig. 16) [77]. It may also occur following diagnostic procedures such as discography, and even myelography. It is usually secondary to intraoperative or intraprocedural contamination and the causative organisms are usually Staphylococcus epidermidis or Staphlococcus aureus. Early diagnosis and treatment is essential in reducing the chances for severe sequelae. However, the MR imaging diagnosis of infectious spondylitis in the postoperative patient is more challenging than in the unoperated patient. Proper diagnosis often relies on a combination of clinical, laboratory, and imaging findings, and often is confirmed through biopsy and culture. Van Goethem and coworkers [77] compared the MR imaging findings in 6 patients with biopsy or surgically proven spondylodiscitis with 38 asymptomatic postoperative patients. They found that contrast enhancement and signal changes in the intervertebral disc or the vertebral endplates were present in postoperative patients who had discitis, but were also seen in asymptomatic patients. However, the absence of Modic type I changes, of contrast enhancement of the disc, or of enhancement of the paravertebral soft tissues suggests that the patient does not have spondylodiscitis. They concluded that the MR imaging appearance was more useful for exclusion than for confirmation of spondylodiscitis [77].

Advances in imaging

Diffusion-weighted imaging

With regard to distinguishing benign from malignant compression fractures, use of plain film is limited by sensitivity. Bone scans and conventional MR sequences are sensitive for the detection of compression fractures, but may be nonspecific in defining the cause. This diagnostic dilemma has given rise to the creation of new techniques for evaluation.

Traditionally, diffusion weighting has been used widely for detection of cerebral ischemic disease [78]. However, within the last 10 years, diffusion-weighted imaging has been studied increasingly as a potential technique for differentiating benign osteoporotic compression fractures from those caused by malignant neoplastic disease. Unfortunately, T2-weighted and STIR sequences do not differentiate intracellular water signal intensity of malignant disease from the interstitial water signal of fracture edema. Diffusion-weighted sequences use these differences for characterization of tissue pathology. Diffusion-sensitizing gradients theoretically cause free extracellular water in fractures to dephase, leading to a loss of signal, whereas the intracellular restricted water within a tumor-infiltrated vertebral

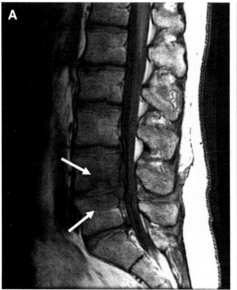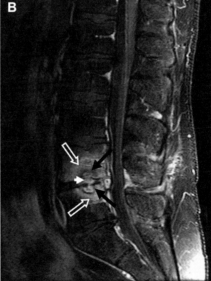

Fig. 16. Postmicrodiskectomy infectious spondylitis. (*A*) Sagittal T1-weighted MR image of the lumbar spine and (*B*) sagittal T1-weighted MR image obtained of the lumbar spine after intravenous administration of gadolinium demonstrate abnormal edema (*white arrows in A and B*) and enhancement in the L4 and L5 vertebral bodies (*open white arrows in B*) and intervertebral disc (*white arrowhead in B*), with partial destruction of the endplate (*black arrows*). This patient presented with recurrent back pain 6 weeks after microdiskectomy.

body should remain in phase (Fig. 17) [79]. Malignant compression fractures typically demonstrate increased signal intensity on diffusion-weighted images, whereas benign compression fractures remain hypointense [79,80]. Diffusion-weighted imaging may also be of use in follow-up of malignant spine disease for treatment response, because a decrease in diffusion signal intensity may correlate with clinical improvement [81]. However, pathologic fractures may still contain a mixture of interstitial extracellular and neoplastic intracellular water [82]. It has been shown that diffusion-weighted imaging can be positive, even in benigndisease [83,84]. Also, diffusion-weighted imaging in the spine can be difficult technically because of the magnetic susceptibility variation and physiologic motion around the spine [85]. These factors may be overcome with the use of line scan and single-shot, fast-spin echo diffusion imaging [85,86]. At this time, diffusion-weighted imaging remains controversial for spine imaging and is still of questionable usefulness.

The usefulness of diffusion-weighted imaging for discriminating infectious spondylitis from malignancy has also been discussed, because the appearance on conventional MR can often overlap. It is well-known that intracranial abscess formation often can show restricted diffusion in comparison with brain tumors. However, the apparent diffusion coefficient values for malignancy and infection may overlap significantly, thus limiting diffusion-weighted imaging's usefulness in the spine [87].

Chemical shift

Chemical shift imaging relies on the differences in precessional frequencies between fat and water. Within a voxel containing both fat and water, signal is dependent on the time of echo and resonance frequencies of the two populations. At a time of echo of 4.2 ms, the resonance frequencies of both fat and water are in phase, and signal contributions from both are additive. However, at 2.1 ms and 6.3 ms, the spins are out of phase and the signal drops out when both fat and water are contained within the same voxel, forming the basis for the evaluation of admixture lesions, such as fatty infiltration of the liver or adrenal adenomas. Normal bone marrow should contain an admixture of fat and water, and signal is expected to decrease within vertebral bodies on out-of-phase images. When fat-containing mature bone marrow becomes replaced or infiltrated, signal may not decrease as expected (Fig. 18). Therefore, chemical shift imaging may be useful in detecting the presence of signal abnormality in the vertebral bone marrow and may aid in differentiating benign from malignant compression fractures. Because visual detection of signal dropout may be limited, regions of interest may help to quantify. Zajick and coworkers [88] have proposed a 20% decrease in signal intensity as an indicator of normal bone marrow. The in- and out-of-phase technique may also be useful in monitoring the response of the tumor to treatment [89].

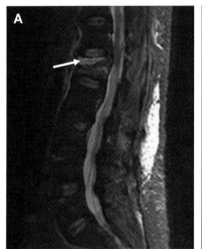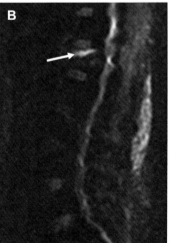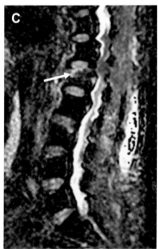

Fig. 17. Benign compression fracture. (*A*) Sagittal fat-saturated T2-weighted MR image of the lumbar spine, (*B*) diffusion-weighted MR image of the lumbar spine, and (*C*) Apparent Diffusion Coefficient map of the lumbar spine demonstrate edema in the superior aspect of the L1 vertebral body with partial collapse (*white arrow in A*). Diffusion-weighted images (*white arrow in B*) and ADC map (*white arrow in C*) showed high signal intensity only in the area corresponding to regions of increased T2 signal intensity (T2 shine through), which suggested that the cause of the compression fracture was benign and not caused by infection or underlying malignancy.

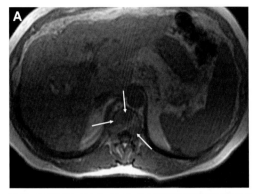

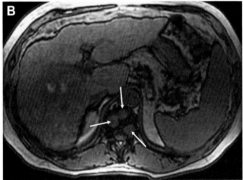

Fig. 18. Metastatic colon carcinoma. (*A*) Axial in-phase MR image and (*B*) axial out-of-phase MR image obtained at the level of the lower thoracic spine show multiple lesions in a thoracic spine vertebral body that have intermediate signal intensity on the in-phase sequence and do not have significant signal drop-out on the out-of-phase sequences (*white arrows in A and B*), suggesting that the lesions did not contain significant fat as would normal marrow. These characteristics suggest malignancy and may be seen in metastatic disease.

Unfortunately, despite its ability to detect abnormal marrow, it cannot distinguish replacement by neoplastic versus nonneoplastic processes [90].

Summary

The spinal marrow has a varied imaging appearance based on the patient's age, and can be affected by diffuse processes ranging from degenerative disc disease to metastatic malignancy. Infectious, inflammatory, metabolic, and neoplastic marrow processes can have a similar appearance on standard T1-weighted, T2-weighted, and STIR MR imaging sequences. The use of intravenous contrast agents, novel imaging techniques such as diffusion-weighted, and in- and out-of-phase imaging can help optimize diagnostic accuracy. These techniques, combined with a careful evaluation of the distribution of the marrow abnormalities, the morphologic appearance of the vertebral body, and the paraspinal tissues, further increases diagnostic accuracy. Ultimately, MR imaging evaluation of the marrow can help avoid unnecessary biopsies in cases of benign processes, and can help determine which patients would benefit from a percutaneous biopsy or a follow-up examination.

References

[1] Ricci C, Cova M, Kang YS, et al. Normal age-related patterns of cellular and fatty bone marrow distribution in the axial skeleton. Radiology 1990;177:83–8.

[2] Modic MT, Steinberg PM, Ross JS, et al. Degenerative disk disease: assessment of changes in vertebral body marrow with MR imaging. Radiology 1988;166:193–9.

[3] Stevens SK, Moore SG, Kaplan ID. Early and late bone-marrow changes after irradiation: MR evaluation. AJR Am J Roentgenol 1990;154:745–8.

[4] Kaplan PA, Helms CA, Dussault R, et al. Musculoskeletal MRI. Philadelphia: WB Saunders Company; 2001. p. 23–53.

[5] Foon KA, Rai KR, Gale RP. Chronic lymphocytic leukemia: new insights into biology and therapy. Ann Intern Med 1990;113:525–39.

[6] Rozman C, Montserrat E. Chronic lymphocytic leukemia. N Engl J Med 1995;333:1052–7.

[7] Han T, Barcos M, Emrich L, et al. Bone marrow infiltration patterns and their prognostic significance in chronic lymphocytic leukemia: correlations with clinical, immunologic, phenotypic, and cytogenetic data. J Clin Oncol 1984;2: 562–70.

[8] Lecouvet FE, Vande Berg BC, Michaux L, et al. Chronic lymphocytic leukemia: changes in bone marrow composition and distribution assessed with quantitative MRI. J Magn Reson Imaging 1998;8:733–9.

[9] Schweitzer ME, Levine C, Mitchell DG, et al. Bull's eyes and halos: useful MR discriminators of osseous metastases. Radiology 1993;188: 249–52.

[10] Friedman DP. Symptomatic vertebral hemangiomas: MR findings. AJR Am J Roentgenol 1996; 167:359–64.

[11] de Roos A, Kressel H, Spritzer C, et al. MR imaging of marrow changes adjacent to end plates in degenerative lumbar disk disease. AJR Am J Roentgenol 1987;149:531–4.

[12] Toyone T, Takahashi K, Kitahara H, et al. Vertebral bone-marrow changes in degenerative lumbar disc disease: an MRI study of 74 patients with low back pain. J Bone Joint Surg Br 1994; 76:757–64.

[13] Mitra D, Cassar-Pullicino VN, Mccall IW. Longitudnal study of vertebral type-1 endplate changes on MR of the lumbar spine. Eur Radiol 2004;14:1574–81.

[14] Kuisma M, Karppinen J, Niinimaki J, et al. Modic type and lumbar level affects painfulness of modic changes. Presented at the Annual Meeting of the International Society for the Study of the Lumbar Spine. New York, May 10–14, 2005.

[15] Grive E, Rovira A, Capellades J, et al. Radiologic findings in two cases of acute Schmorl's nodes. AJNR Am J Neuroradiol 1999;20:1717–21.

[16] Dagirmanjian A, Schils J, McHenry MC. MR imaging of spinal infections. Magn Reson Imaging Clin N Am 1999;7:525–38.

[17] Mahboubi S, Morris MC. Imaging of spinal infections in children. Radiol Clin North Am 2001;39:215–22.

[18] Khan IA, Vaccaro AR, Zlotolow DA. Management of vertebral discitis and osteomyelitis. Orthopedics 1999;22:758–65.

[19] Tins BJ, Cassar-Pullicino VN. MR imaging of spinal infection. Semin Musculoskelet Radiol 2004; 8:215–29.

[20] Varma R, Lander P, Assaf A. Imaging of pyogenic infectious spondylodiscitis. Radiol Clin North Am 2001;39:203–13.

[21] Ratcliffe JF. Anatomic basis for the pathogenesis and radiologic features of vertebral osteomyelitis and its differentiation from childhood discitis. Acta Radiol Diagn (Stockh) 1985;26(2): 137–43.

[22] Sapico FL. Microbiology and antimicrobial therapy of spinal infections. Orthop Clin North Am 1996;27:9–13.

[23] Longo M, Granata F, Ricciardi GK, et al. Contrast-enhanced MR imaging with fat suppression in adult-onset septic spondylodiscitis. Eur Radiol 2003;13:689–94.

[24] Ledermann HP, Schweitzer ME, Morrison WB, et al. MR imaging findings in spinal infections: rules or myths. Radiology 2003;228:506–14.

[25] Joseffer SS, Cooper PR. Modern imaging of spinal tuberculosis. J Neurosurg Spine 2005;2: 145–50.

[26] Ahmadi J, Bajaj A, Destian S, et al. Spinal tuberculosis: atypical observations at MR imaging. Radiology 1993;189:489–93.

[27] Moorthy S, Prabhu NK. Spectrum of MR imaging findings in spinal tuberculosis. AJR Am J Roentgenol 2002;179:979–83.

[28] Jung N, Jee W, Ha K, et al. Discrimination of tuberculous spondylitis from pyogenic spondylitis on MRI. AJR Am J Roentgenol 2004;182: 1405–10.

[29] Krishnan A, Patkar D, Patankar T, et al. Craniovertebral junction tuberculosis: a review of 29 cases. J Comput Assist Tomogr 2001;25:171–6.

[30] Narlawar RS, Shah JR, Pimple MK, et al. Isolated tuberculosis of posterior elements of spine: magnetic resonance imaging findings in 33 patients. Spine 2002;27:275–81.

[31] Harman M, Unal O, Onbasi KT, et al. Brucellar spondylodiscitis MRI diagnosis. Clin Imaging 2001;25:421–7.

[32] Rotes-Querol J. Osteo-articular sites of brucellosis. Ann Rheum Dis 1957;16:63–8.

[33] Spink WW. The nature of brucellosis. Minneapolis (MN): University of Minnesota Press; 1956.

[34] Kurugoglu S, Kanberoglu K, Kanberoglu A, et al. MRI appearances of inflammatory vertebral osteitis in early ankylosing spondylitis. Pediatr Radiol 2002;32:191–4.

[35] Romanus R, Yden S. Destructive and ossifying spondylitic changes in rheumatoid ankylosing spondylitis. Acta Orthop Scand 1952;22:88–99.

[36] Stanitski CL. Conditions of the spine. Adolesc Med 1998;9:515–32.

[37] Sadat-Ali M, Ammar A, Corea JR, et al. The spine in sickle cell disease. Int Orthop 1993;18:154–6.

[38] Reynolds J. A re-evaluation of the "fish vertebra" sign in sickle cell hemoglobinopathy. AJR Am J Roentgenol 1966;97:693–707.

[39] Marlow TJ, Brunson CY, Jackson S, et al. "Tower vertebra": a new observation in sickle cell disease. Skeletal Radiol 1998;27:195–8.

[40] Resnik CS, Young JW, Aisner SC, et al. Case report 594. Skeletal Radiol 1990;19:79–81.

[41] Ginsberg LE, Williams DW, Stanton C. MRI of vertebral sarcoidosis. J Comput Assist Tomogr 1993;17:158–9.

[42] Le Breton C, Ferroir JP, Cadranel J, et al. Case report 825. Skeletal Radiol 1994;23:297–300.

[43] Fisher AJ, Gilula LA, Kyriakos M, et al. MR imaging changes of lumbar vertebral sarcoidosis. AJR Am J Roentgenol 1999;173:354–6.

[44] Poyanli A, Poyanli O, Sencer S, et al. Vertebral sarcoidosis: imaging findings. Eur Radiol 2000; 10:92–4.

[45] Shaikh S, Soubani AO, Rumore P, et al. Lytic osseous destruction in vertebral sarcoidosis. N Y State J Med 1992;9:213–4.

[46] Lisle D, Mitchell K, Crouch M, et al. Sarcoidosis of the thoracic and lumbar spine: imaging findings with an emphasis on magnetic resonance imaging. Australas Radiol 2004;48:404–7.

[47] Archibeck MJ, Rosenberg AG, Sheinkop MB, et al. Gout-induced arthropathy after total knee arthroplasty: a report of two cases. Clin Orthop 2001;392:377–82.

[48] Fenton P, Young S, Prutis K. Gout of the spine. Two case reports and a review of the literature. J Bone Joint Surg Am 1995;77:767–71.

[49] Chang I. Surgical versus pharmacologic treatment of intraspinal gout. Clin Orthop Relat Res 2005;433:106–10.

[50] Miller LJ, Pruett SW, Losada R, et al. Clinical image. Tophaceous gout of the lumbar spine: MR findings. J Comput Assist Tomogr 1996;20: 1004–5.

[51] Feydy A, Liote F, Carlier R, et al. Cervical spine and crystal-associated diseases: imaging findings. Eur Radiol 2006;16:459–68.

[52] Dudler J, Stucki RF, Gerster JC. Aseptic psoas pyomyositis and erosive discitis in a case of calcium pyrophosphate crystal deposition disease. Rheumatology (Oxford) 2000;39:1290–2.

[53] Poll LW, Koch JA, vom Dahl S, et al. Type I Gaucher disease: extraosseous extension of skeletal disease. Skeletal Radiol 2000;29:15–21.

[54] Hermann G, Shapiro RS, Abdelwahab IF, et al. MR imaging in adults with Gaucher disease type I: evaluation of marrow involvement and disease activity. Skeletal Radiol 1993;22: 247–51.

[55] Blocklet D, Abramowicz M, Schoutens A. Bone, bone marrow, and MIBI scintigraphic findings in Gaucher's disease "bone crisis". Clin Nucl Med 2001;26:765–9.

[56] Katz K, Mechlis-Frish S, Cohen J, et al. Bone scan in the diagnosis of bone crisis in patients who have Gaucher disease. J Bone Joint Surg Am 1991;73:513–7.

[57] Katz K, Sabato S, Horev G, et al. Spinal involvement in children and adolescents with Gaucher disease. Spine 1993;18:332–5.

[58] Fox H, McCarthy P, Andre-Schwartz J, et al. Gaucher's disease and chronic lymphocytic leukemia. Cancer 1984;54:312–4.

[59] Shiran A, Brenner B, Laor A, et al. Increased risk of cancer in patients with Gaucher disease. Cancer 1993;72:219–24.

[60] Rosenthal DI, Barton NW, McKusick KA, et al. Quantitative imaging of Gaucher disease. Radiology 1992;185:841–5.

[61] Vande Berg BC, Malghem J, Devuyst O, et al. Anorexia nervosa: correlation between MR appearance of bone marrow and severity of disease. Radiology 1994;193:859–64.

[62] Old JL, Calvert M. Vertebral compression fractures in the elderly. Am Fam Physician 2004; 69:111–6.

[63] Tehranzadeh J, Tao C. Advances in MR imaging of vertebral collapse. Semin Ultrasound CT MR 2004;25:440–60.

[64] Jensen ME, Evans AJ, Mathis JM, et al. Percutaneous polymethylmethacrylate vertebroplasty in the treatment of osteoporotic vertebral body compression fractures: technical aspects. AJNR Am J Neuroradiol 1997;18:1897–904.

[65] Irani FG, Morales JP, Sabharwal T, et al. Successful treatment of a chronic post-traumatic 5-year-old osteoporotic vertebral compression fracture by percutaneous vertebroplasty. Br J Radiol 2005;78:261–364.

[66] Kaufmann TJ, Jensen ME, Schweickert PA, et al. Age of fracture and clinical outcomes of percutaneous vertebroplasty. AJNR Am J Neuroradiol 2001;22:1860–3.

[67] Tanigawa N, Komemushi A, Kariya S, et al. Percutaneous vertebroplasty: relationship between vertebral body bone marrow edema pattern on MR images and initial clinical response. Radiology 2006;239:195–200.

[68] Mathis JM. Percutaneous vertebroplasty: complication avoidance and technique optimization. AJNR Am J Neuroradiol 2003;24:1697–706.

[69] Mathis JM, Barr JD, Belkoff SM, et al. Percutaneous vertebroplasty: a developing standard of care for vertebral compression fractures. AJNR Am J Neuroradiol 2001;22:373–81.

[70] Stallmeyer MJB, Zoarski GH, Obuchowski AM. Optimizing patient selection in percutaneous vertebroplasty. J Vasc Interv Radiol 2003;14: 683–96.

[71] Voormolen MHJ, van Rooij WJ, van der Graaf Y, et al. Bone marrow edema in osteoporotic vertebral compression fractures after percutaneous vertebroplasty and relation with clinical outcome. AJNR Am J Neuroradiol 2006;27:983–8.

[72] Dansie DM, Luetmer PH, Lane JI, et al. MRI findings after successful vertebroplasty. AJNR Am J Neuroradiol 2005;26:1595–600.

[73] Trout AT, Kallmes DF, Kaufmann TJ. New fractures after vertebroplasty: adjacent fractures occur significantly sooner. AJNR Am J Neuroradiol 2006;27:217–23.

[74] Uppin AA, Hirsch JA, Centenera LV, et al. Occurrence of new vertebral body fracture after percutaneous vertebroplasty in patients with osteoporosis. Radiology 2003;226:119–24.

[75] Grados F, Depriester C, Cayrolle G, et al. Long-term observations of vertebral osteoporotic fractures treated by percutaneous vertebroplasty. Rheumatology (Oxford) 2000;39:1410–4.

[76] Lin EP, Ekholm S, Hiwatashi A, et al. Vertebroplasty: cement leakage into the disc increases the risk of new fracture of adjacent vertebral body. AJNR Am J Neuroradiol 2004;25:175–80.

[77] Van Goethem JWM, Parizel PM, van den Hauwe L, et al. The value of MRI in the diagnosis of postoperative spondylodiscitis. Neuroradiology 2000;42:580–5.

[78] Moseley ME, Cohen Y, Mintorovitch J, et al. Early detection of regional cerebral ischemia in cats: comparison of diffusion- and T2-weighted MRI and spectroscopy. Magn Reson Med 1990;14: 330–46.

[79] Spuentrup E, Buecker A, Adam G, et al. Diffusion-weighted MR imaging for differentiation of benign fracture edema and tumor infiltration of the vertebral body. AJR Am J Roentgenol 2001; 176:351–8.

[80] Baur A, Huber A, Ertl-Wagner B, et al. Diagnostic value of increased diffusion weighting of a steady-state free precession sequence for differentiating acute benign osteoporotic fractures from pathologic vertebral compression fractures. AJNR Am J Neuroradiol 2001;22:366–72.

[81] Byun WM, Shin SO, Chang Y, et al. Diffusion-weighted MR imaging of metastatic disease of the spine: assessment of response to therapy. AJNR Am J Neuroradiol 2002;23:906–12.

[82] LeBihan D, Turner R, Douek P, et al. Diffusion MR imaging: clinical applications. AJR Am J Roentgenol 1992;159:591–9.

[83] Castillo M. Diffusion-weighted imaging of the spine: is it reliable? AJNR Am J Neuroradiol 2003;24:1251–3.

[84] Castillo M, Arelaez A, Smith JK, et al. Diffusion-weighted MR imaging offers no advantage over

routine noncontrast MR imaging in the detection of vertebral metastases. AJNR Am J Neuroradiol 2000;21:948–53.

[85] Bammer R, Herneth A, Maier SE, et al. Line scan diffusion imaging of the spine. AJNR Am J Neuroradiol 2003;24:5–12.

[86] Park SW, Lee JH, Ehara S, et al. Single shot fast spin echo diffusion-weighted MR imaging of the spine: is it useful in differentiating malignant metastatic tumor infiltration from benign fracture edema? Clin Imaging 2004;28:102–8.

[87] Pui MH, Mitha A, Rae WID, et al. Diffusion-weighted magnetic resonance imaging of spinal infection and malignancy. J Neuroimaging 2005;15:164–70.

[88] Zajick DC, Morrison WB, Schweitzer ME, et al. Benign and malignant processes: normal values and differentiation with chemical shift MR imaging in vertebral marrow. Radiology 2005;237:590–6.

[89] Erlya WK, Oha ES, Outwater EK. The utility of in-phase/opposed-phase imaging in differentiating malignancy from acute benign compression fractures of the spine. AJNR Am J Neuroradiol 2006;27:1183–8.

[90] Disler DG, McCauley TR, Ratner LM, et al. In-phase and out-of-phase MR imaging of bone marrow: prediction of neoplasia based on the detection of coexistent fat and water. AJR Am J Roentgenol 1997;169:1439–47.

MAGNETIC
RESONANCE
IMAGING CLINICS

Magn Reson Imaging Clin N Am 15 (2007) 199–219

MR Imaging Evaluation of the Bone Marrow and Marrow Infiltrative Disorders of the Lumbar Spine

Faisal Alyas, FRCR, Asif Saifuddin, FRCR, David Connell, FRANZCR*

The lumbar spine has important roles in structural support and in facilitating normal truncal movement. It is part of our mineral store and is active in hematopoiesis throughout life. Bone marrow diseases frequently affect areas that are hematopoietically active. The most common of the disease processes that affect the bone marrow is metastatic disease. MR imaging of the lumbar spine is performed most frequently to characterize degenerative spinal disease using T1-weighted (T1W) and T2-weighted (T2W) imaging sequences. MR imaging, with its excellent contrast resolution, is also highly sensitive in detecting [1–6], but less specific [7–9] in diagnosing, inflammatory disease and benign and malignant bone marrow involvement. It now has a well-established role in the imaging of bone marrow disease, particularly in staging the disease and in guiding biopsy [8–16].

Imaging of bone marrow disease requires a good understanding of the composition, function, and range of appearances of normal bone marrow and the changes that occur with increasing age and increasing hematopoietic demand. An appreciation is also required of the contemporary imaging sequences currently used, including T1W spin echo (SE), short tau inversion recovery (STIR), in- and out-of-phase gradient echo (GRE), and diffusion-weighted sequences, and some of the techniques that are used to modify these sequences, including fat suppression and contrast enhancement. Finally, the wide range of infiltrative disease processes affecting this tissue also needs to be understood. These processes can be divided into disorders that affect the hematopoietic and reticulin components, and changes that occur secondary to treatment for marrow disorders. Diseases of the

Department of Radiology, Royal National Orthopaedic Hospital, Brockley Hill, Stanmore, Middlesex, London, UK, HA7 4LP
* Corresponding author.
E-mail address: david.connell@rnoh.nhs.uk (D. Connell).

doi:10.1016/j.mric.2007.03.002
mri.theclinics.com

hematopoietic component can be divided further into those that cause replacement, proliferation, or depletion of this component. Diseases of the reticulin component of marrow include mastocytosis and myelofibrosis. Changes secondary to treatment can result from chemotherapy, radiation, and granulocyte colony–stimulating factor (GCSF). These disease processes are discussed in this article. The authors do not review diseases of bone mineralization and bone loss (eg, Paget's disease, osteoporosis) or red cell dysplasias of the hematopoietic marrow (eg, sickle cell disease) because these processes are beyond the scope of this article.

Function and composition of lumbar vertebral marrow

Marrow is one of the largest organs in the body, consisting of two components named after gross histologic findings. Red marrow, which is hematopoietically active, is found mainly in the axial skeleton, and yellow marrow, which is largely hematopoietically inactive, mostly occupies the peripheral skeleton [17]. Red marrow and yellow marrow are not entirely homogeneous and each contains elements of the other.

The lumbar vertebrae contain marrow that is mostly red marrow, and have a surrounding thin rim of cortical bone and a central framework of predominantly vertically orientated trabeculae. The osseous portion has structural function, contains stores of phosphate and calcium, and acts as a support framework for the cellular components. Production of blood cells is the most important function of vertebral marrow. The various blood cells are derived from pluripotential stem cells that develop into erythroid cells (red blood cells), granulocytes, monocytes (macrophages), thrombocytes (platelets), and lymphoid cells (lymphocytes). Marrow also contains reticulum cells, consisting of phagocytic and nonphagocytic cells, including macrophages and fibroblasts, and sparse fat cells, although many fewer than in yellow marrow. These cells may have a function in nutritional support and in providing growth factors for hematopoietic cells [1]. A rich sinusoidal supply is derived from vessels that pierce the cortex. One or two large basivertebral veins drain the vertebrae posteriorly into Batson's plexus. Nerves run along with these vessels, and lymph nodes can be identified within the marrow [1]. The vertebral marrow is a dynamic organ that changes with age, immune status, oxygenation, coagulation status, and structural needs.

Imaging sequences

The signal returned by normal marrow depends on the balance of fat to cellular components within the marrow [8]. The red marrow in vertebra contains predominantly hematopoietic cells (60% hematopoietic and 40% fat cells) and, hence, returns signal related to both fat and water. In comparison, yellow marrow is predominantly fat-containing (95% fat cells and 5% hematopoietic cells) [18], which returns signal following fat. The balance changes with increasing fat component (conversion from red marrow to yellow marrow) and age, and according to sex, as described later. In addition, some changes are related to reconversion from yellow marrow to red marrow as a result of increased hematopoietic demand. The net result is heterogeneous and variable signal from red marrow in normal lumbar vertebrae, along with possible areas of focal red and yellow marrow change and progressive age-related fatty replacement of red marrow. Because marrow disease can appear similar to red marrow, the distinction between the two can be difficult to make [8,17]. Fortunately, in the elderly, the predominant signal intensity follows fat in vertebral marrow and makes distinction from disease possible, particularly on T1W and fat-suppressed sequences.

The trabecular network contributes to the decreasing signal from marrow by creating magnetic field inhomogeneities at the trabecular/cellular interface, particularly on gradient recalled echo (GRE) sequences. The reduction in trabecular bone with increasing age may account in part for the increasing signal with aging on these sequences.

Sequences that detect changes in the water/fat distribution, the trabeculae, edema, cell density, and marrow vascularity can help identify the presence of marrow disease [9]. Although T2W sequences are less sensitive for the detection of marrow disease, the appearances of abnormalities are described because this sequence is used commonly in lumbar spine imaging.

T1-weighted spin echo

T1W SE sequences are the workhorse of bone marrow imaging [1]. Adult red marrow returns an intermediate signal that is higher than intervertebral disc or muscle, which is related to complex and poorly understood interactions between equal quantities of fat and water, together with a smaller contribution from a protein component [10,17]. Any signal lower than the associated muscle or intervertebral disc is abnormal. Yellow marrow normally follows fat signal, appearing hyperintense because of the short T1 relaxation time of fat. Trabeculae contribute little to signal because of the 180° rephasing gradient in these SE sequences [8,17].

Fat saturation and short tau inversion recovery sequences

STIR imaging uses an inversion pulse of varying time to cancel signal from fat. This pulse also reduces signal from other short T1 relaxation substances such as blood and contrast. Disadvantages include a relatively long imaging time and chemical shift artifact. Because of the high sensitivity of STIR, if lesions are undetected on this sequence, then further imaging or contrast enhancement (for the purpose of lesion detection) may be unnecessary [19].

Fat saturation sequences selectively null signal from fat using a presaturation pulse and do not reduce signal from areas with similar relaxation time. These sequences are particularly useful in diminishing the signal contribution from fat and in improving the dynamic contrast range. Normal marrow on a T1W contrast-enhanced sequence can be difficult to distinguish from abnormal marrow, which displays marked enhancement, because both return high signal intensity. This contrast enhancement may cause increased signal in the regions of otherwise decreased signal occupied by abnormal marrow. This phenomenon occasionally can decrease the conspicuity of metastases on contrast-enhanced sequences. Abnormal contrast enhancement is also seen more easily with fat suppression.

On fat-saturated sequences, red marrow has intermediate-to-high signal intensity (the intermediate is similar to muscle), depending on the degree of cellularity, and yellow marrow appears hypointense. Marrow disease usually produces increased signal on STIR or other fluid-sensitive sequences and on contrast-enhanced sequences [8,17,20–22].

Gradient recalled echo and in- and out-of-phase imaging (chemical shift imaging)

On GRE sequences, the trabecular bone component normally results in reduced signal of normal marrow because of the tendency to produce susceptibility artifact and the normally low level of signal produced by mature bone. Infiltration of bone marrow resulting in trabecular destruction can increase signal on this sequence, which may be of use in detecting infiltrative marrow disease and in assessing the degree of involvement (ie, to determine the risk of pathologic fracture) [23].

In- and out-of-phase, or chemical shift, imaging is particularly useful for differentiating focal red marrow from tumor, which takes advantage of two facts: the resonance frequencies of water and fat are different; and normal red marrow and some benign diseases have a fat/water ratio that is approximately equal to, or greater than, one. The signal of marrow on GRE imaging depends on the timing of the refocusing echo pulse. If timed so that the fat and water phases are aligned (in-phase), the signal intensities are summed, whereas if they are completely out-of-phase, they subtract. Normal red marrow and benign fatty-containing lesions (normal vertebral end plate degeneration, Schmorl's nodules with edema, hemangiomas, benign fractures) lose signal on chemical shift imaging and therefore return low signal on the out-of-phase imaging sequence [24]. Hypercellular marrow disease, however, shows either no change or an increase in signal intensity [11,25].

Some investigators have found that a greater than 20% signal drop-off is significantly predictive of benign disease, whereas signal increase or no drop-off implies malignancy [24,26]. Yellow marrow remains unchanged but can be distinguished on the basis of signal that follows fat [10,25].

The main disadvantage is that appearances of benign hematopoietic, but hypercellular, marrow and marrow disease overlap somewhat, particularly if the marrow abnormality is detected early. This technique has also been used to quantify the volume of fat in hematopoietic malignancies and in other benign marrow infiltrative disorders such as Gaucher's disease. This quantification may be used for treatment planning and in monitoring the effectiveness of the prescribed treatment.

Diffusion-weighted imaging

Diffusion-weighted imaging was first described in the brain for distinguishing tumors from infarction. In bone marrow, it has been used most frequently to differentiate between benign and malignant fractures of the vertebral bodies.

Benign fractures have interstitial edema that has less restricted diffusion (thereby giving rise to low signal or signal that is isointense to the surrounding vertebral body). Malignant fractures, on the other hand, contain intracellular water from cell infiltration in combination with some interstitial edema and therefore demonstrate restricted diffusion (high signal on the diffusion-weighted images). Long imaging times can limit its use because of motion artifact, a possible problem for patients who are attempting to stay motionless while suffering significant pain from a vertebral fracture [27,28]. Imaging techniques, such as obtaining the diffusion-weighted imaging with echoplanar imaging, may reduce artifacts by decreasing imaging time [29]. Other benign disease, such as edema related to infection and treated metastatic disease, may be differentiated effectively from neoplasia by diffusion-weighted imaging [29].

Differing degrees of cellularity (hypocellular, normocellular, hypercellular) can be distinguished by detecting the degree of diffusion restriction, which may be useful in differentiating subtle marrow disease from normal marrow. Detecting an increase in diffusion produced by necrotic cells following chemotherapy may also be a useful way of monitoring the effects of the chemotherapy [29].

Contrast enhancement

Normal adult red and yellow marrow displays no significant enhancement with gadolinium that can be appreciated by the naked eye on T1W images [17]. However, a measurable signal difference of 15% can be detected when the interstices of the marrow are measured [30–32]. Marrow disease tends to enhance markedly and it is essential to compare postcontrast images with the unenhanced precontrast images because it may be difficult to distinguish marrow disease from normal high signal marrow on T1W images [8]. Significant enhancement of highly cellular marrow can be found in infants and children in the first few years of life [33].

Dynamic imaging has been used to assess disease status and for treatment follow-up. Normal marrow shows a decrease in maximal enhancement, slope of enhancement, and washout time with increasing age and fat content [31,32]. Lymphoma and myeloma both have an increased slope, maximum enhancement, and reduced washout over time, in comparison with age-matched normal marrow [34].

Enhancement with novel agents such as iron oxide can be useful in distinguishing hypercellular marrow from the abnormal marrow that may be seen in such scenarios as metastases, lymphoma, and posttreatment changes (eg, after GCSF). The superparamagnetic iron oxide is taken up and metabolized by hematopoietic cells of the reticuloendothelial system, resulting in negative enhancement with T1, T2, and STIR imaging. Tumor cells do not take up iron oxide, resulting in no signal loss [35]. The regions affected by tumor therefore demonstrate increased signal in a background of decreased signal produced by the normal uptake of the iron oxide.

Heterogeneity of normal lumbar vertebral marrow signal

The normal adult lumbar spine contains mainly red marrow that appears as intermediate signal on T1W images (Fig. 1). This signal within the marrow is normally higher than that of the adjacent intervertebral disc. On T2 fat saturated sequences, the marrow typically has intermediate to moderately high

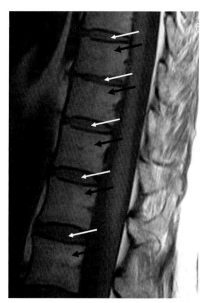

Fig. 1. Normal marrow. A 31-year-old woman with a history of back pain demonstrates normal marrow. Sagittal T1W SE (echo time [TE] 14, repetition time [TR] 480) image shows uniform bone marrow (*black arrows*) with intermediate signal greater than that of the intervertebral disc (*white arrows*).

signal intensity [36]. The marrow composition and signal intensity are also different, depending on the sex. Men have a minimally increased fat content compared with that of women and therefore have relatively increased signal on T1W images and decreased signal on T2W images with fat saturation [37]. As the patient ages, the marrow assumes a more variable appearance with the progressive increase in fat content and reduction in red cell mass and trabecular/cortical bone [8,10,11,17]. The changes that occur with aging are part of the normal process of conversion from red marrow to yellow marrow.

Conversion predominately affects the peripheral skeleton and results in a progressive transfer of red marrow to yellow marrow in a symmetric, distal-to-proximal manner [8,10,17]. The vertebra, however, tends to maintain its red marrow content until relatively late. At birth, the vertebra is entirely red marrow and is predominantly cellular, but becomes progressively fatty with increased age (Fig. 2) [38]. Thus, the vertebral marrow in infants and children demonstrates low signal (lower than muscle) on T1W (see Fig. 2A) and increases in signal with age, to the point where it has greater signal than the nearby muscle. The normal adult marrow signal of the vertebral bodies is greater than that of muscle and intervertebral disc on the T1W images. The adult signal intensity of the bone

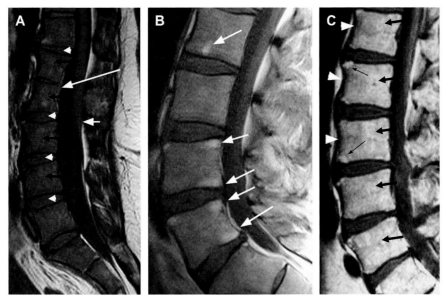

Fig. 2. Normal marrow changes with age. (*A*) A 14-year-old boy with a history of diastematomyelia, failure of segmentation of L2/L3, and normal marrow. Sagittal T1W SE (echo time [TE] 15, repetition time [TR] 490) image demonstrates normal marrow signal for age (*black arrows*), which appears almost the same signal as intervertebral disc (*white arrowheads*). The fused L2/L3 vertebrae (*long white arrow*) and low-lying conus (*short white arrow*) are demonstrated. (*B*) A 20-year-old man with normal marrow. Sagittal T1W SE (TE 15, TR 500) image demonstrates intermediate signal marrow higher than the signal of the child in Fig. 2A. In addition, focal areas of increased marrow signal are demonstrated, primarily in the regions subjacent to the vertebral end plates (*arrows*). (*C*) A 60-year-old man with normal marrow. Sagittal T1W SE (TE 14, TR 500) image demonstrates a diffuse high signal, consistent with normal marrow (*large black arrows*). The more hematopoietic marrow predominates in the anterior portion of the vertebral body (*white arrowheads*). Again, fatty marrow is seen in the anterior vertebral bodies adjacent the end plates (*small black arrows*).

marrow is usually reached by 30 years of age (see Fig. 1) [1,10].

One of the factors contributing to the increase in the fatty component of marrow with age is that a common precursor gives rise to osteoblasts and adipocytes. An increased adipogenesis with age, therefore, may lead to a decreased osteoblastogenesis [10,39,40]. These areas of increased fatty deposition within the red marrow are most predominant in the posterior elements (Fig. 3A), along the basivertebral veins, and in bands along the end plates (see Fig. 2B, C). The latter is caused by ischemia, ageing, or degeneration of adjacent discs [41,42]. The red marrow in vertebrae predominates at the metaphyseal equivalents near the superior and inferior end plates [17,41] and at the anterior portions of the vertebral bodies (see Fig. 2C) [36]. These changes tend to occur in all vertebrae in a similar way and in symmetric fashion.

Focal areas of fat deposition can occur as part of the process of conversion. The focal areas can occur anywhere in the vertebrae although, as mentioned, the focal fat tends to be deposited in the posterior elements, along the end plates, and around the basivertebral plexus [36,41,43].

Focal areas of red marrow deposition are also possible [11,17,29] and these may have a focal area of fat centrally (Fig. 3B). This focal region of central fat is a result of the normal centrifugal direction of marrow conversion. During red marrow reconversion (and after bone marrow transplantation) a similar process occurs but in a centripetal direction [44]. A fuzzy peripheral border is seen with earlier conversion, whereas a sharper border is seen in the more advanced stages. These areas tend to occur peripherally within the vertebrae, to have a symmetric distribution, to be parallel to subchondral bone, and to have an elongated shape [17,36,45]. Diffusion-weighted imaging can be used to distinguish between these focal areas of red marrow and neoplastic marrow disease.

In normal spinal marrow, these patterns of fatty and hematopoietic marrow distribution result in various signal changes. Ricci and colleagues [41] categorized these into four main patterns of marrow distribution: (1) uniform low signal with high linear signal around the basivertebral vein (Fig. 4A); (2) band-like high signal limited to the periphery of the vertebral body (see Fig. 3A; Fig. 4B); (3) multiple small indistinct (and difficult to visualize)

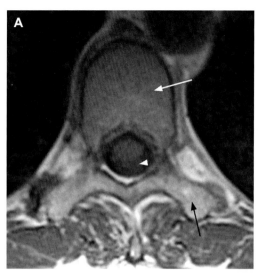
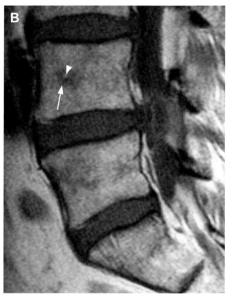

Fig. 3. Normal marrow in the posterior elements and bull's eye sign. (*A*) A 35-year-old woman with a meningioma and normal marrow. Axial T1W SE (echo time [TE] 15, repetition time [TR] 450) image demonstrates normal marrow signal in the vertebral body (*white arrow*) that is lower than the marrow in the posterior elements (*black arrow*). The meningioma is also seen posterior to the spinal cord (*arrowhead*). (*B*) A 50-year-old man with lower back pain, demonstrating a normal bull's eye sign. Sagittal T1W SE (TE 20, TR 570) image through the L4 vertebral body shows a normal focus of low signal hematopoietic marrow (*arrow*) and a focus of high fat signal in the center of the red marrow (*arrowhead*).

high signal foci (a few millimeters across) throughout the vertebral body (see Fig. 3B; Fig. 4C); and (4) multiple larger high signal foci (5–15 mm) throughout the vertebral body (Fig. 4D). A combination of the first and last two types was also identified. Pattern 1 is increasing in frequency in the younger age group (<30 years old), with a growing frequency of patterns 2 and 3 with increasing age. Most of the type 1 pattern occurs in those under 30 years old and most of the type 2 and 3 patterns occur in those more than 40 years old. The second type was not seen in the thoracic spine, probably is related to mechanical stresses in the spine, and is not present to the stabilizing effect of the ribs or related to degenerative disc changes [41,42].

These variations should be considered when assessing marrow for disease. In addition, other sequences, such as low signal on out-of-phase GRE images and intermediate or low signal intensity on fat-suppressed images (see Fig. 4D), can be used to confirm benign marrow, rather than disease.

Infiltrative marrow diseases

Infiltrative marrow diseases are categorized best according to the manner in which the marrow is altered. These diseases can result in proliferation,

replacement, depletion, or dysplasia of normal marrow components. Infiltrative marrow disease can be classified further on the basis of the component of marrow that is affected: hematopoietic cells or the reticulum. Important changes can also be recognized in hematopoietic marrow, as a result of various types of treatment. These treatments include radiograph therapy for neoplastic disorders, chemotherapy, and GCSF (given for individuals with a decreased white blood cell count). Generally, marrow infiltrative disease produces a low signal on the T1W images and high signal on the fluid-sensitive sequences because of the reduced fat and increased water content [10]. Most of these cases are metastases and, in the older patient who has more fatty vertebral marrow, the metastatic disease is typically very conspicuous on the T1W images. In the younger patient, more diffuse infiltrative disorders are more common, and may have low or intermediate signal changes on the T1W images that are similar to red marrow, possibly making the distinction from normal hematopoietic marrow difficult.

Metastases tend to cause multifocal involvement, whereas other infiltrative disease tends to present in a more diffuse pattern. Three main patterns of marrow involvement are common: focal involvement,

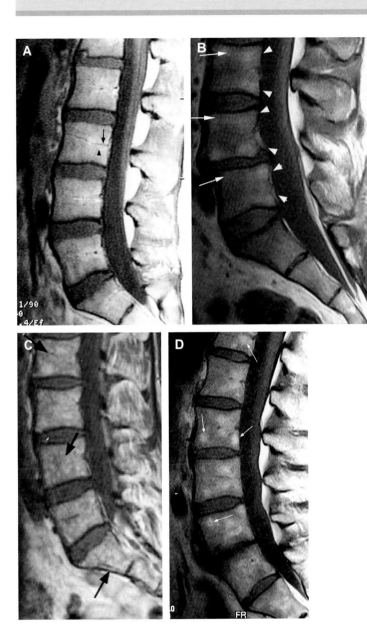

Fig. 4. Normal patterns of fatty distribution according to Ricci. (*A*) A 39-year-old man with type 1 normal marrow. Sagittal T1W SE (echo time [TE] 15, repetition time [TR] 550) image demonstrates linear low signal (*black arrow*) surrounded by linear high signal (*arrowhead*). (*B*) A 39-year-old woman with grade 1 degenerative spondylolisthesis and type 2 marrow. Sagittal T1W SE (TE 15 TR 540) image demonstrates symmetric low signal in the metaphyseal equivalent just below the end plates (*arrows*). Bandlike and triangular areas of fatty marrow replacement are in the periphery of the vertebral body (*arrowheads*). (*C*) A 60-year-old woman with back pain demonstrating type 3a normal marrow patterns. Sagittal T1W SE (TE 15, TR 550) image shows multiple small foci of high fatty signal (*black arrows*) superimposed on a background of intermediate signal hematopoietic marrow. (*D*) A 36-year-old woman with a degenerate L4/L5 disc and normal type 3b fatty marrow. Sagittal T1W SE (TE 16, TR 540) image demonstrates multiple, relatively large areas of fatty bone marrow (*white arrows*).

seen in the solitary case of primary bone tumors and plasmacytoma; multiple focal lesions, seen frequently in metastasis, myeloma, and myelodysplasia; and diffuse disease, seen in proliferative and replacement disorders such as myeloma, leukemia, and non-Hodgkin's lymphoma. A normal marrow appearance can occasionally be identified in early lymphocyte and plasma cell malignancies and in some cases of high-grade myeloma and acute myeloid leukemia (AML). These patterns are not exclusive to any particular disease process, and different patterns may affect different vertebrae. The areas of abnormal signal do not always correlate with abnormal biopsy results, which is a consequence of the potentially similar appearances of neoplastic

marrow infiltration and normal hypercellular hematopoietic marrow that may proliferate in response to disease [11].

Overall, MR imaging may not always be able to distinguish among the different disease processes, but it has an increasing role in identifying the burden of disease, helping stratify the treatment options, and monitoring response in a noninvasive way.

Proliferation

Benign proliferation can result in normal proliferation of red marrow caused by physiologic changes as part of the normal response to alterations in hematopoietic demand. This process is red marrow reconversion. Abnormal proliferation of the normal components of bone marrow may be caused by myelodysplasia, polycythemia, leukemia, myelomas, or amyloidosis. Because these disease processes affect the cellular components of marrow and are usually diffuse, they may be difficult to distinguish from normal red marrow when the disease burden is low. Here, more advanced imaging techniques, such as chemical shift imaging and contrast enhancement, may be useful in distinguishing the two.

Marrow reconversion

When hematopoietic demand increases, marrow undergoes red marrow reconversion, with hyperplasia of red marrow elements. The vertebral bodies are the first to be affected in this process and these fatty areas revert to a more cellular marrow. An expansion of the marrow space and an increase in the cellularity of any islands of red marrow may also be seen [10,46]. Normally, this finding can be seen, to a mild degree, in smokers, the obese, and marathon runners as increased marrow MR imaging signal on the fluid-sensitive sequences and decreased signal on T1W images [47,48]. More prominent marrow changes with very high signal on the fluid-sensitive sequences and low signal on the T1W images are seen in chronic disease and diffuse marrow pathology (eg, anemias, hematopoietic malignancies), and as a consequence of chemotherapy, radiotherapy, or GCSF [49]. Relatively new contrast agents using negative enhancement with iron oxide show promising results in distinguishing benign red marrow reconversion from neoplastic infiltration.

Multiple myeloma

Multiple myeloma is classified as a plasma cell dyscrasia and can present as a diffuse infiltration of plasma cells or as focal disease (known as a plasmacytoma). The plasma cell dyscrasias frequently affect the hematopoietic-rich axial skeleton and result in a monoclonal proliferation of atypical plasma cells. Myeloma can be graded histologically, depending on the degree of plasma cell infiltration. The plasma cell infiltration is reported as a percentage of the total marrow cell mass. The percentage of plasma cells in myeloma is typically reported as low (10% to 20%), intermediate (20% to 50%) or high (>50%). The disease may also be staged by designating it stage 1, 2, or 3, according to the staging system of Durie and Salmon. Typically, this classification system was applied based on the serum hemoglobin, serum calcium, radiograph appearance of the osseous structures, M-gradient on electrophoresis, and urine Bence-Jones protein levels. Recently, a simplified version of the criteria has been proposed, using serum albumin and beta 2-microglobulin. As the stage and grade of the disease increases, the corresponding survival rate decreases. The stage and grade are useful in selecting the specific treatment [50]. The main uses of MR imaging are in defining and staging the disease, establishing the prognosis, and quantifying the patient's response to treatment.

Monoclonal gammopathy of undetermined significance (MGUS) is a potentially premalignant disease, which is characterized by an abnormal amount of a single immunoglobin in the blood. Most remain asymptomatic but up to 30% of these patients may progress to a more aggressive form of the disease, even up to 25 years after the initial discovery of the monoclonal gammopathy. The more advanced forms of the disease include amyloidosis, Waldenstrom's macroglobulinemia, and multiple myeloma [51]. The MGUS can be difficult to distinguish from asymptomatic myeloma on laboratory studies alone. MR imaging studies are normal in MGUS [50,52] but abnormal, by one report, in 31% of asymptomatic myeloma [50,53,54].

Five different patterns of infiltration may be identified on MR imaging, including a normal-appearing marrow, focal infiltration, diffuse disease, variegated involvement, or combined neoplastic infiltration of multiple myeloma. A normal appearance of the bone marrow may occur in approximately 28% of cases and is seen as high signal on the T1W images and intermediate-to-low T2W signal on the fat-suppressed sequences. The normal marrow appearance corresponds to less than 20% marrow infiltration [55]. This appearance tends to occur more frequently in low-grade disease and MGUS, but may also occur in more advanced stages (up to stage 3 disease) [56].

Up to 30% of cases have shown focal area of disease corresponding to low or isointense signal on the T1W images and are poorly visualized on the T2W images because of signal similar to marrow fat [55]. These focal lesions may be visualized best on fat-suppressed or chemical shift imaging sequences as regions of increased signal (Fig. 5A, B) [57,58].

Diffuse bone marrow involvement results in low signal on T1W sequences and is usually the result of moderate- to high-grade disease. When high-grade disease is present, the T1W signal can be almost the same as that of the intervertebral discs but with more moderate grades, the marrow may have a similar signal to that of normal marrow (Fig. 5C) [55]. In patients older than 30, enhancement of more than 40% of the baseline signal is consistent with malignant infiltration. This enhancement pattern is seen most often with intermediate- to high-grade disease because low-grade

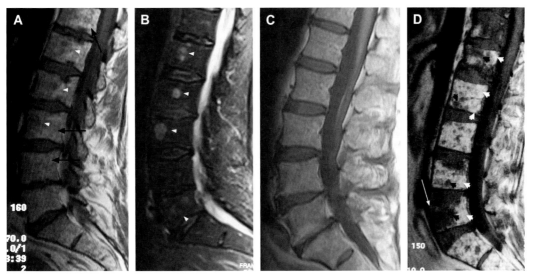

Fig. 5. Myeloma. (*A* and *B*) A 43-year-old man with moderate-grade myeloma demonstrating focal disease and diffuse disease. (*A*) Sagittal T1W SE (echo time [TE] 15 repetition time [TR] 580) sequence shows diffuse patchy increased signal (*black arrows*). These areas show no high signal on the fat saturated T2W fast SE (TE 80, TR 4500) sequence (*B*) and are consistent with fatty marrow. The subtle focal areas of low signal on T1W are more conspicuous as high signal on fat saturated images (*white arrowheads* in *A* and *B*). Different patterns of disease can coexist, which can be consistent with myeloma infiltration and part of the spectrum of the variegated pattern of infiltration. (*C*) A 45-year-old man with low-grade myeloma. Sagittal T1W SE (TE 20, TR 600) images demonstrate very subtle diffuse lowering of marrow signal that is difficult to distinguish from normal marrow. In early disease, infiltration may be insufficient to cause marrow signal change. Fatty marrow elements may also proliferate. (*D*) A 46-year-old woman with variegated multiple myeloma. Sagittal T1W SE (TE 15, TR 500) image demonstrates multiple small foci of low signal (*black arrowheads*) and separate larger foci of high signal (*white arrowheads*) from fatty marrow. These areas have the classic variegated appearance of myeloma. Further larger areas of low signal (*white arrow*) may also be seen. In a relatively young woman, such diffuse increase in signal should raise the possibility of secondary aplastic anemia.

disease most often does not enhance much more than normal marrow [59].

The variegated, or salt-and-pepper, appearance occurs in approximately 3% of patients, most often in those patients who have low-grade disease. The abnormal plasma cells may also stimulate the release of hematopoiesis-inhibiting factor by the tumor cells, resulting in multiple small foci of high signal on T1W sequences (corresponding to fat islands) within a background of low signal caused by plasma cell infiltration. The regions of tumor involvement typically are seen as regions of decreased signal on the T1W images and increased signal on the T2W images (see Fig. 5A; Fig. 5D). Typically, no hypointensity will be seen on the fat-suppressed imaging sequences in the regions of tumor involvement in the patients with this variegated appearance (see Fig. 5B, D) [55,60].

Eleven percent of patients have combined diffuse and focal disease (see Fig. 5). All forms of the disease may also have a background of hematopoietic change, which can cause further lowering of the signal on the T1W images as a result of red marrow reconversion.

The grade of infiltration has been shown to correlate with the degree of enhancement of marrow. The mean level of contrast enhancement from baseline has been reported as 18% in the control group, 26% in patients who had low-grade infiltration, 49% in patients who had intermediate-grade infiltration, and 90% in patients who had high-grade infiltration. This level is related directly to the degree of cellular involvement and microvessel content and inversely to the fat content of marrow [61].

The frequency of abnormalities detected by MR imaging depends also on the stage of disease. MR imaging can detect disease in 25% to 50% of cases of low-grade disease. In high-grade lesions, the rate of detection improves to more than 80% [54,62,63].

MR imaging is also useful in determining the progression of early disease. MR imaging detection of disease in asymptomatic stage 1 disease myeloma and MGUS is correlated with earlier onset of more aggressive disease [53,63]. Imaging staging combined with clinical staging may be more useful in determining survival than either alone. Diffuse and multiple focal involvement have a worse survival prognosis compared with variegated and normal-appearing bone marrow (as demonstrated on MR imaging) [64]. Extent of disease may be more important in determining prognosis than focal and diffuse pattern of involvement [64]. The pattern of involvement and detection of involvement in high-grade disease may also be useful in determining response to treatment. Lecouvet and colleagues found better response to treatment in stage 3 disease, compared with those with no detectable disease on MR imaging in the spine. Diffuse disease was also noted to be associated with worse clinical disease in this cohort of patients [57].

The response to treatment can also be assessed with diffuse disease changing to variegated or focal disease, and moderate enhancement decreasing to minimal enhancement. A complete response results in marrow signal returning to normal with no abnormal enhancement or peripheral enhancement [65]. A popular current staging system for myeloma (by Durie and Salmon) includes a modification using MR imaging and fludeoxyglucose F 18–positron emission tomography (FDG-PET) imaging findings, with an increasing number of focal lesions and increasingly diffuse disease classified as higher-grade disease (Table 1) [50].

Waldenstrom's macroglobulinemia

Waldenstrom's macroglobulinemia is a rare, low-grade lymphoid cell malignancy characterized by production of monoclonal immunoglobin and the infiltration of lymph nodes, the spleen, and the bone marrow. Up to 19% of patients may progress to a more aggressive form of the monoclonal gammopathy up to 10 years after the initial discovery of disease. This progression can require additional treatment and it is important to identify this subsegment of patients early so the appropriate treatment can be initiated. Imaging findings similar to the diffuse and variegated patterns of myeloma have been described for patients who have Waldenstrom's macroglobulinemia, but focal lesions have not been described. Abnormal MR imaging findings may be seen in 91% to 100% of patients, and a direct association has been found between a decreased level of enhancement and a positive clinical response [66,67].

Amyloidosis

Amyloidosis is a rare disease that can occur in isolation (primary amyloidosis) or may be familial [68]. Amyloidosis may also occur as a result of chronic disease, either inflammatory or neoplastic. Most of the cases of amyloidosis previously seen have been in patients undergoing hemodialysis with old blood filter types that failed to remove β2 microglobin. This failure resulted in the deposition of β2 microglobin and resultant destructive spondyloarthropathy or diffuse systemic deposition [69,70]. Diffuse low signal on both T1 and T2W sequences has been described in both the primary [71] and secondary forms [72].

Leukemia

The leukemias are a heterogeneous group of conditions arising from malignant proliferation of white cells. The acute subtypes, including AML and acute lymphoid leukemia, result from the growth of immature cells and occur frequently in children. The chronic subtypes, including chronic myeloid leukemia (CML) and chronic lymphoid leukemia, result from overgrowth of mature cells and frequently occur in the elderly. Diagnosis is based on examination of peripheral blood smears and bone marrow biopsy. As with the other proliferative disorders, these conditions most commonly will have diffusely low signal on T1W MR images [1,9,10,73–75], but, with some forms of leukemia, the bone marrow may have a normal appearance in approximately 10% of patients (ie, with AML) [76]. Other methods of diagnosing leukemias include using chemical shift GRE sequences, proton spectroscopy, and bulk T1 relaxation techniques. These techniques have been found to show marrow involvement with greater consistency [77–79].

MR imaging also has a role in determining prognosis and in following the course of treatment.

Table 1: Modification of the Durie and Salmon "PLUS" staging system of myeloma using MR imaging and fludeoxyglucose F 18–positron emission tomography

Classification[a]	Whole-body MR imaging or fludeoxyglucose F 18–positron emission tomography
MGUS	All negative
Stage I A	Normal skeletal survey or single lesion (smoldering)
Stage I B	<5 focal lesions or mild diffuse disease
Stage II A/B	5–20 focal lesions or moderate diffuse disease
Stage III A/B	>20 focal lesions or severe diffuse disease

[a] Subclassification in stages II and III: A, normal renal function; B, abnormal renal function.

One study demonstrated a worse prognosis with prolonged bulk T1 relaxation time in early CML [74]. Measurement of bulk T1 relaxation of marrow can also give an estimate of the quantity of regenerating marrow and can therefore provide an estimate of treatment success [77,80]. Larger series have indicated that this measurement is of more value in acute lymphoid leukemia than AML [79,81], and may be related to the longer T1 relaxation lymphoid cells [82]. It may reduce the need for obtaining repeat biopsies when following the treatment of acute leukemias. Dynamic contrast enhancement may also provide a means of monitoring response by assessing degree and rate of contrast uptake. Contrast uptake primarily depends on cellularity and vascularity of the marrow [34,83]. Measurement of the degree of contrast enhancement of the marrow can also help to identify remission and relapse and identify the presence of new disease.

Polycythemia vera

Polycythemia vera is an idiopathic proliferation of pluripotential stem cells, particularly involving the erythrocytic cell line [10]. Typically, the MR imaging appearance is characterized by diffuse homogenous reduction in signal on T1W images, consistent with hypercellularity. This appearance may be difficult or impossible to distinguish from other hematologic malignancies [9]. A more focal pattern of replacement is also possible [84]. Fifteen percent of cases undergo postpolycythemic myeloid metaplasia. The proliferation decreases over time and the hypercellular marrow is replaced by fibrosis, resulting in myelofibrosis, which usually appears low signal on all sequences [10,84].

Replacement disorders

The following diseases are the most common infiltrative marrow diseases and result from replacement of normal marrow with cells that are not inherent to normal bone marrow.

Metastasis

Metastasis is certainly the most common lesion to affect the vertebral marrow, particularly in those over 40 years of age. The rich blood supply to the red marrow predisposes to metastases, particularly in the vertebral column [85]. It is well established that MR imaging is more sensitive for detecting metastasis than other imaging modalities [86–88].

The most common primary tumors that metastasize to the spine are prostate tumors and breast tumors. Most are osteolytic (breast, bronchus, kidney, thyroid) and return high signal on the fluid-sensitive sequences, and are detected as low signal (classically lower than disc in the lumbar spine) on the T1W images. Osteoblastic metastasis (prostate, breast, transitional cell carcinoma, carcinoid) may appear hypointense on both the T1W images and the fluid-sensitive images. Mixed metastases can occur in breast and lung (and more rarely in other malignancies such as prostate or lymphoma), giving a heterogeneous appearance (Fig. 6A, B). Melanoma is unusual in that it can return high signal on T1 (Fig. 6C) and T2/STIR sequences. All metastases can enhance markedly with contrast. On dynamic contrast-enhanced imaging, malignant lesions attain a rapid peak enhancement and wash out early. Benign lesions, on the other hand, can have persistent enhancement for up to 10 minutes [23].

Morphologically, metastases are usually more focal (Fig. 6D), in comparison with the diffuse involvement of proliferative marrow disease. The posterior elements can be involved, although the body of the vertebra is affected most frequently (see Fig. 6D). The incidence of cortical destruction is greater than with hematologic malignancies [89]. The pedicles may be the first area of destruction and tumor tends not to extend beyond the end plate because of the barrier effect caused by the end plate and intervertebral disc (see Fig. 6B). Halos of high STIR/T2W signal, consistent with mucinous or cellular tissue in the leading edge of trabecular destruction, are suggestive of malignant disease (see Fig. 6B) [44]. A more diffuse pattern occurs less frequently, compared with the hematologic malignancies, occurring more so in the vertebral body (Fig. 6E) [89].

The distinction between benign (osteoporotic, traumatic) and malignant vertebral fractures can be difficult with both having similar features of low signal on T1W and high signal on T2W and fat suppressed imaging [90]. Some features, such as fracture lines, lack of extension into the pedicles or posterior elements, lack of a soft tissue mass, and the preservation of some normal T1 fat signal within the vertebral body, may help to delineate benign from malignant fractures.

Features associated with malignant fractures include multifocal involvement with signs of metastasis elsewhere, infiltration and edema of the posterior elements [91], a convex posterior vertebral body border (see Fig. 6A, C), soft tissue mass, and well-defined tumor margin [23]. Benign fractures tend to preserve fatty marrow signal and have linear fracture lines that may appear sharp or fragmented [90,92]. Benign fractures may also have an angled posterior border or a ruptured disc that is associated with the traumatic fracture [23]. Diffuse high signal within the vertebral body, along with a linear area of higher signal on STIR imaging, is significantly associated with benign osteoporotic fractures [93].

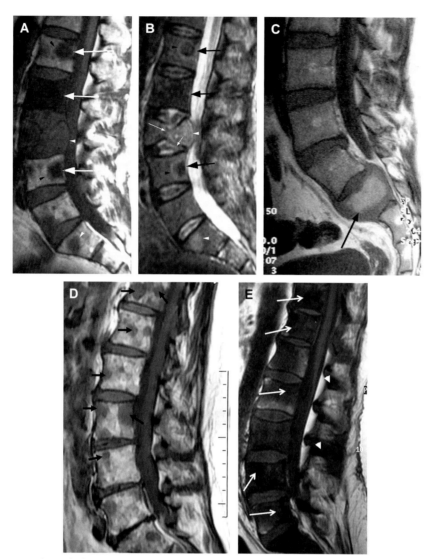

Fig. 6. Metastasis. (*A* and *B*) A 69-year-old man with a history of lytic and sclerotic metastases from prostate cancer. (*A*) Sagittal T1W SE (echo time [TE] 15, repetition time [TR] 530) and (*B*) sagittal T2W fat saturated images (TE 130 TR 5600) demonstrate focal areas of low signal on T1 and T2 images, consistent with sclerotic disease (*large white arrows and black arrowheads*). Additional focal areas of low T1 and high T2 signal are seen consistent with lytic disease (*white arrowheads*). The L3 vertebral body has undergone fracture (*long white arrow*) and is causing spinal stenosis. The intervertebral disc (*short white arrow*) is not involved. Halos (as seen around the lesions in the L1 and L4 vertebral bodies) of high T2 signal are suggestive of malignant disease (*black arrowheads*). (*C*) A 44-year-old woman with a history of melanoma. Sagittal T1W SE (TE 15, TR 550) images show a slightly expansile high signal mass replacing the S1 vertebral body (*arrow*). The biopsy results from this region were consistent with melanoma metastasis. (*D*) A 70-year-old woman with a history of metastatic lung cancer. Sagittal T1W SE (TE 12, TR 530) image demonstrates multiple focal areas of low signal (*black arrows*) consistent with metastasis. Other diseases, including high-grade lymphoma and myeloma, may appear similar. (*E*) A 78-year-old man with a history of prostate cancer. Sagittal T1W SE (TE 12, TR 530) image demonstrates diffuse low marrow signal within the vertebral bodies (*white arrows*) and within the posterior elements (*white arrowheads*), consistent with diffuse metastatic infiltration.

At 1 to 3 months, marrow signal usually reverts to normal or becomes increased because of fatty replacement on the T1W images [90].

Some levels within the lumbar spine may be affected more frequently by metastatic fractures than by benign fractures. One study suggested that the incidence of metastatic fractures in L5 (12 of 51 cases) was significantly different than that of fractures of the L1 level (4 of 51) in age-matched controls [94].

Diffusion-weighted imaging has shown its usefulness at distinguishing benign from malignant fractures [27,28,95]. One study has shown a specificity of 93% and a positive predictive value of 91% [96]. Malignancy shows restricted diffusion appearing as having increased signal on diffusion-weighted sequences (see previous section).

Lymphoma

Most bony lymphomatous involvement results from hematogenous spread (95%) and rarely as primary bone marrow disease. It occurs more commonly in those with non-Hodgkin's (20% to 40%) than Hodgkin's (5%) disease [10,97–99]. The most common pattern is a diffuse, mottled pattern of disease that typically occurs with lower grade lymphomas (Fig. 7). Multiple focal areas of involvement typically occur in Hodgkin's and less frequently in high-grade non-Hodgkin's lymphomas [8]. Large soft tissue masses, which can encase bone and cause permeative bone destruction without cortical destruction, are usually seen in primary, rather than secondary, lymphoma [100]. Most commonly, MR imaging signal is reduced on T1 and T2W sequences, although the signal is usually more variable on the T2W sequences (see Fig. 7). Intense areas of high signal on T2W and STIR imaging may

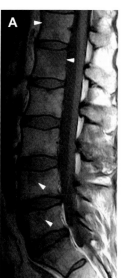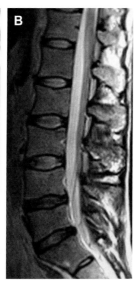

Fig. 7. Lymphoma. A 35-year-old man with a history of low-grade lymphoma. (*A*) Sagittal T1W SE (echo time [TE] 14, repetition time [TR] 570) and (*B*) sagittal T2W images (TE 140, TR 5000) demonstrate diffuse areas of patchy low signal intensity on the T1W images (*white arrowheads* in *A* and *B*) that are not visible on the T2W images. The disease process that produces this appearance gives rise to low signal on both sequences. This appearance is consistent with diffuse low-grade disease infiltration.

occur in nodular sclerosing forms of Hodgkin's disease, and are thought to represent an immature fibrotic reaction [10]. Reduced signal in the lumbar spine on T1W images is also associated with an increased relapse rate in patients who have had Hodgkin's disease [101].

MR imaging is useful in detecting disease when biopsy is negative [102] and in guiding biopsy, thus decreasing the possibility for sampling error from a blind biopsy [99]. In addition, MR imaging has advantages in measuring disease burden and in detecting sites of normal marrow for harvesting autologous transplantation marrow [103].

Depletion

Depletion results in a reduction of normal red marrow volume in a distribution and quantity more than accepted with normal physiologic changes, and occurs as a consequence of aplastic anemia and treatments such as chemotherapy and radiotherapy.

Aplastic anemia and myelodysplastic syndrome

Aplastic anemia results in pancytopenia and can be produced by a number of different causes. These include idiopathic causes (which are though to be autoimmune), metastatic disease, leukemia, infections, organic solvents, reaction to drugs (gold, phenylbutazone, and chloramphenicol), after hepatitis, and as a predictable reaction to cancer treatments (see later discussion). Most aplastic anemias, however, have no known cause [10]. A diffuse depletion of red marrow and replacement with acellular fatty marrow may be seen. The fatty marrow replacement is most striking in areas of normal high red marrow concentration such as the spine, but may be difficult to detect in areas with predominately fatty marrow such as the appendicular skeleton [104].

Approximately 30% to 60% of patients who have aplastic anemia improve following treatment with steroids or immunosuppressive therapy [10]. After treatment, focal islands of red marrow may be identified as part of a red marrow reconversion process. These islands can be hypercellular hematopoietic marrow, but can simulate other disease processes such as myelodysplasia and other preleukemic conditions that can occur in chronic aplastic anemia [65]. In chronic aplastic anemia, a significant proportion of patients progress to myelodysplasia or preleukemic disease. In approximately one third of cases, myelodysplasia can transform to leukemia [9]. Various patterns suggest transformation, including focal areas of low signal, more inhomogeneous signal, and diffuse cellular patterns [106]. STIR imaging and contrast-enhanced imaging may be useful in distinguishing between red marrow reconversion and transformation of aplastic anemia (ie, on STIR imaging, myelodysplasia can appear as heterogeneously high signal) [56,104]. Treatment of these conditions may result in a uniformly marginally high signal on STIR imaging [104].

A novel, dynamic, contrast-enhanced technique using chemical shift imaging has been shown to distinguish between normal marrow, aplastic anemia, myelodysplastic syndrome, and other diffuse marrow disease (ie, polycythemia and CML). This method uses a chemical shift misregistration technique to isolate the water portion of marrow from the fat portion. The contrast enhancement of the water component showed a lower peak value for aplastic anemia and a higher contrast peak value for myelodysplasia, compared with normal marrow, CML, and polycythemia. The washout of contrast in patients who had aplastic anemia was also comparatively slower [105].

Reticulum

Myelofibrosis

Myelofibrosis can result from the same spectrum of disease as polycythemia but can also be related to infection, metastatic disease, or Gaucher's disease, or it may have no definite cause and be designated as idiopathic. Increasing fibrosis results in diffuse low signal on all sequences (Fig. 8A) and hypercellularity has also been reported, thereby making it

sometimes difficult to distinguish myelofibrosis from other infiltrative marrow diseases [9,10,84, 106]. The extent of the involvement of marrow fibrosis may be useful in evaluating the clinical prognosis, because increasing marrow fibrosis is associated with more severe anemia or pancytopenia and a worsening of the prognosis [107].

Systemic mastocytosis

Systemic mastocytosis is part of the spectrum of mastocytosis that includes systemic and leukemic mastocytosis. It results from an abnormal proliferation of mast cells that accumulate in the skin, bone marrow, spleen, liver, and lymph nodes. Bones are involved in 70% of cases, with the spine being affected most frequently [108]. Other myeloproliferative and myelodysplastic syndromes may be associated with it [109,110]. Mast cell proliferation in the bone marrow results in a fibroblastic and granulomatous reaction that typically causes trabecular destruction and new bone formation [111]. Histamine release results in calcium deposition, but prostaglandin release may cause osteopenia [110]. The result is diffuse or focal osteopenia or osteosclerosis [9] which, on T1W and SITR/T2W sequences, results most often in diffuse low signal, reflecting medullary sclerosis (Fig. 8B, C) [112]. Low signal on the T1W images [9,108] and high signal on the fluid-sensitive sequences, or intermediate signal on T1W and the fluid-sensitive sequences,

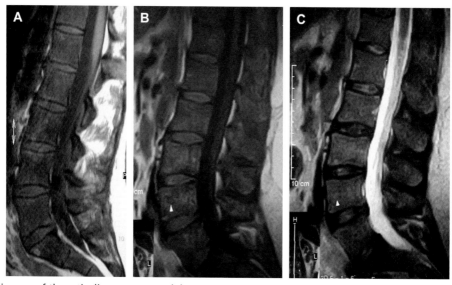

Fig. 8. Diseases of the reticulin component. (*A*) A 67-year-old man with a history of myelofibrosis. Sagittal T1W SE (echo time [TE] 14, repetition time [TR] 470) image demonstrates diffuse low signal throughout all vertebral bodies. This finding is nonspecific, occurring in many other diseases, including mastocytosis, lymphoma, Gaucher's disease, and, rarely, metastatic disease. (*B* and *C*) A 30-year-old male patient with a history of mastocytosis. (*B*) Sagittal T1W SE (TE 15, TR 530 and (*C*) sagittal T2W images (TE 130 TR 5600) demonstrate diffuse low signal on both sequences, consistent with diffuse infiltration. More focal areas of low signal T1 and intermediate signal T2 can also be seen (*white arrowheads*), which may represent more focal disease.

have also been demonstrated [110]. Although classically a diffuse homogenous low signal infiltration has been described, reticular, mottled, or normal/inhomogeneous patterns of disease infiltration may occur in one half of all cases [108,110,113]. These patterns, however, are not associated with any particular subtype of disease or any specific findings seen on the biopsy specimens [108,110].

Metabolic/miscellaneous

Hemosiderin deposition

Hemosiderin can be deposited in bone marrow macrophages, caused by chronic breakdown of blood products in chronic hemolytic anemias, repeated transfusions, acquired immunodeficiency syndromes, or metabolic conditions such as hemochromatosis, and can result in very low signal on all sequences and possibly blooming artifact on GRE imaging [114].

Lysosomal storage disorders

Gaucher's disease is the most common of these rare conditions and results from absence of the enzyme glucocerebroside hydrolase, which results in accumulation of the glycolipid glucosylceramide in histiocytes and subsequent fibrosis throughout the reticuloendothelial system. The lumbar spine is one of the first sites of involvement [115] and the site of marrow involvement generally follows the distribution of red marrow [1]. Complications from the diffuse infiltration of bone marrow with glucosylceramide include infarction and osteonecrosis [116]. MR imaging commonly shows diffuse low signal on T1W and T2W sequences (Fig. 9) [115]. Acute disease, however, can have increased signal on T2W images, which can create a diagnostic dilemma because it could be confused with other processes such as infection, infarction, or fracture [117]. Typical morphologic features, such as vertebra plana and platyspondyly, may also appear at multiple levels. Distinguishing normal marrow from diseased marrow may be difficult in young patients [115], and contrast enhancement with iron superoxide may be of value to detect subtle disease in this patient population.

Treatment is with enzyme supplements, and monitoring requires assessment of disease burden with MR imaging [118].

Treatment-related changes

Radiotherapy

In the lumbar spine, marrow changes occur after treatment of diseases such as metastases and myeloma, and as part of bone marrow transplantation. Radiation changes affect the portion of the lumbar pine or sacrum in the region where the radiation field is applied and will have a well-defined cut-

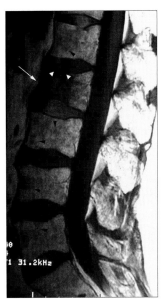

Fig. 9. Gaucher's disease. A 35-year-old man with a history of Gaucher's disease. Sagittal T1W SE (echo time [TE] 14, repetition time [TR] 550) image demonstrates heterogeneous low signal (*white arrowheads*). A more focal area of low signal may be seen (*white arrow*), along with some degree of superior end plate collapse (*white arrowheads*). This superior end plate collapse probably represents a mild superior end plate compression fracture.

off zone between the native marrow and the radiation-treated marrow. Initially after radiation therapy, edema, vascular congestion, and capillary injury to the small vasculature may occur [119], and within the first 2 weeks, there may be dilation of the sinusoidal spaces and hemorrhage [120]. As the changes become chronic, the hematopoietic cells are replaced by yellow marrow [121].

The earliest changes are those of bone marrow edema, hemorrhage, and the early influx of nonirradiated cells that are detectable as increased signal on the fluid-sensitive sequences and variable signal (increased, isointense, or decreased) on the T1W images [119]. Regions of increased signal seen within 2 weeks on T1W images are likely to represent hemorrhage or, possibly, early fatty replacement [122]. High signal on the T1W images may be caused by fatty replacement and can be seen routinely as early as 3 to 6 weeks following radiation therapy (Fig. 10) [119,122].

Enhancement may occur in the early phase following radiation therapy as the sinusoidal spaces enlarge. In the chronic phase, enhancement is reduced because of decreased vascularity and microcirculation. Scattered radiation can also result in similar, but less marked, changes in marrow outside the direct field [122].

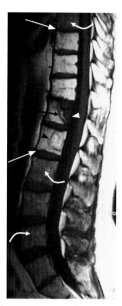

Fig. 10. Radiation. A 42-year-old woman with a history of myeloma treated with radiation. Sagittal T1W SE (echo time [TE] 16, repetition time [TR] 580) image shows the fatty signal change within the limits of the radiation field (*white arrows*). Normal red marrow signal is seen in the vertebrae outside the field (*curved white arrows*). Tumor is identified within the partially collapsed posterior portion of the T12 vertebral body (*white arrowhead*). This vertebra contains a fracture line just anterior to the fracture (*black arrow*). A successfully treated deposit in the L1 vertebra has undergone fatty involution but retains a low signal sclerotic border (*black arrowhead*).

Bone marrow recovery most often occurs between 12 and 24 months following treatment, with patchy red marrow regeneration characterizing the early changes [123]. The degree of recovery depends on the dose given; low doses (<30 Gy) appear to allow full recovery [121], whereas with doses between 30–40 Gy, the red marrow elements have little chance of recovery because of destruction of sinusoids. This is because of the complete destruction of vascular sinusoids which prevent migration of hematopoietic cells [9]. Peripheral bands of low or intermediate signal may also occur and these are thought to represent hematopoietic marrow in the late stage (>6 weeks). These bands are typically seen in younger patients and may reflect their greater ability to recover from the effects of irradiation [119].

Granulocyte colony–stimulating factor

Chemotherapy can cause myeloid cell depletion, resulting in neutropenia. GCSF is a medication that is used as an adjunct to chemotherapy to improve myeloid cell production and function [124].

In red marrow, signal is increased on the fluid-sensitive images and reduced on the T1W images, reflecting red marrow reconversion [125]. Similarly, signal is increased on the out-of-phase GRE imaging and on the T2W or fluid-sensitive images [126,127]. Changes are maximal 2 weeks after administration of the medication and this normal marrow reaction should be distinguished from marrow disease [127]. The changes seen after GCSF administration can mimic diffuse infiltration or, less commonly, focal metastatic disease [126].

Bone marrow transplantation

This technique has been used for the treatment of many conditions, including leukemia and myeloma. MR imaging provides a noninvasive method for identifying normal areas of marrow that may serve as donor sites for bone marrow harvesting and to assess the volume of bone marrow after treatment. Knowledge of the appearance of the typical bone marrow changes seen after transplantation is necessary to interpret appropriately what is observed on posttransplantation imaging. The bone marrow usually undergoes necrosis within the first week, as a result of the ablation, and is seen as having decreased signal on the T1W images and increased signal on the fluid-sensitive (STIR/T2W) images. A bandlike pattern of marrow change most often develops within the vertebral body that has a central high signal corresponding to marrow fat and a peripheral dark signal consistent with repopulating hematopoietic marrow [128,129]. Similarly, on the fluid-sensitive sequences, signal is high initially, followed by reduced signal, followed by peripheral high signal as the marrow reconverts [130]. With successful treatment, the bone marrow then slowly evolves into a more uniform, normal marrow signal.

Summary

The assessment of the appearance of bone marrow disease and of normal marrow requires an understanding of the typical marrow composition seen in both states and the sequences used for imaging. Most infiltrative marrow diseases are not readily distinguished from each other based on the degree and distribution of signal change. The various disease patterns include a normal marrow appearance, a diffuse uniform marrow abnormality, and scattered focal patterns of marrow infiltration (most returning abnormally low signal on the T1W images). Metastatic disease is more commonly multifocal than is nonmetastatic disease. The role of MR imaging is primarily in distinguishing disease from normal marrow. Normal marrow signal does not always exclude subtle marrow infiltrative disease and overlap does occur in the spectrum between normal marrow and marrow disease.

In most cases, the final diagnosis is made based on a combination of the history and laboratory work-up. Occasionally, problem-solving tools include the use of more novel MR imaging sequences such as fat-suppressed imaging, diffusion-weighted imaging, chemical shift imaging, and intravenous contrast enhancement. These techniques can also be used to distinguish benign marrow disease from normal marrow and from malignant disease. MR imaging has a role in establishing prognoses based on the disease pattern and burden of disease. Imaging may also have a role in assessing the patient's response to chemotherapy drugs and to other associated treatments.

References

[1] Vogler JB 3rd, Murphy WA. Bone marrow imaging. Radiology 1988;168(3):679–93.

[2] Pettersson H, Gillespy 1, Hamlin DJ, et al. Primary musculoskeletal tumors: examination with MR imaging compared with conventional modalities. Radiology 1987;164(1):237–41.

[3] Moulopoulos LA, Varma DG, Dimopoulos MA, et al. Multiple myeloma: spinal MR imaging in patients with untreated newly diagnosed disease. Radiology 1992;185(3):833–40.

[4] Smith SR, Williams CE, Davies JM, et al. Bone marrow disorders: characterization with quantitative MR imaging. Radiology 1989;172(3):805–10.

[5] Zimmer WD, Berquist TH, McLeod RA, et al. Bone tumors: magnetic resonance imaging versus computed tomography. Radiology 1985;155(3):709–18.

[6] Avrahami E, Tadmor R, Dally O, et al. Early MR demonstration of spinal metastases in patients with normal radiographs and CT and radionuclide bone scans. J Comput Assist Tomogr 1989;13(4):598–602.

[7] Sugimura K, Yamasaki K, Hajime K, et al. Bone marrow diseases of the spine: differentiation with T1 and T2 relaxation times in MR imaging. Radiology 1987;165(2):541–54.

[8] Vanel D, Dromain C, Tardivon A. MRI of bone marrow disorders. Eur Radiol 2000;10(2):224–9.

[9] Nobauer I, Uffmann M. Differential diagnosis of focal and diffuse neoplastic diseases of bone marrow in MRI. Eur J Radiol 2005;55(1):2–32.

[10] Steiner RM, Mitchell DG, Rao VM, et al. Magnetic resonance imaging of diffuse bone marrow disease. Radiol Clin North Am 1993;31(2):383–409.

[11] Vande Berg BC, Lecouvet FE, Michaux L, et al. Magnetic resonance imaging of the bone marrow in hematological malignancies. Eur Radiol 1998;8(8):1335–44.

[12] Herneth AM, Friedrich K, Weidekamm C, et al. Diffusion weighted imaging of bone marrow pathologies. Eur J Radiol 2005;55(1):74–83.

[13] Ghanem N, Altehoefer C, Hogerle S, et al. Comparative diagnostic value and therapeutic relevance of magnetic resonance imaging and bone marrow scintigraphy in patients with metastatic solid tumors of the axial skeleton. Eur J Radiol 2002;43(3):256–61.

[14] Flickinger FW, Sanal SM. Bone marrow MRI: techniques and accuracy for detecting breast cancer metastases. Magn Reson Imaging 1994;12(6):829–35.

[15] Yao L, Seeger LL. MR effective at detecting pathology of marrow space. Diagn Imaging 1991;13(7):116–20.

[16] Depaoli L, Davini O, Foggetti MD, et al. Evaluation of bone marrow cellularity by magnetic resonance imaging in patients with myelodysplastic syndrome. Eur J Haematol 1992;49(2):105–7.

[17] Vande Berg BC, Malghem J, Lecouvet FE, et al. Magnetic resonance imaging of normal bone marrow. Eur Radiol 1998;8(8):1327–34.

[18] Snyder WS, Cook MJ, Nasset ES, et al. Report of the task group on reference man. In: ICRP, editor. International commission on radiological protection. Oxford (UK): Pergamon Press; 1975. p. 85–98.

[19] Mahnken AH, Wildberger JE, Adam G, et al. Is there a need for contrast-enhanced T1-weighted MRI of the spine after inconspicuous short tau inversion recovery imaging? Eur Radiol 2005;15(7):1387–92.

[20] Simon JH, Szumowski J. Chemical shift imaging with paramagnetic contrast material enhancement for improved lesion depiction. Radiology 1989;171(2):539–43.

[21] Mirowitz SA, Apicella P, Reinus WR, et al. MR imaging of bone marrow lesions: relative conspicuousness on T1-weighted, fat-suppressed T2-weighted, and STIR images. Am J Roentgenol 1994;162(1):215–21.

[22] Mirowitz SA. Fast scanning and fat-suppression MR imaging of musculoskeletal disorders. Am J Roentgenol 1993;161(6):1147–57.

[23] Vanel D, Bittoun J, Tardivon A. MRI of bone metastases. Eur Radiol 1998;8(8):1345–51.

[24] Zajick DC Jr, Morrison WB, Schweitzer ME, et al. Benign and malignant processes: normal values and differentiation with chemical shift MR imaging in vertebral marrow. Radiology 2005;237(2):590–6.

[25] Seiderer M, Staebler A, Wagner H. MRI of bone marrow: opposed-phase gradient-echo sequences with long repetition time. Eur Radiol 1999;9(4):652–61.

[26] Erly WK, Oh ES, Outwater EK. The utility of in-phase/opposed-phase imaging in differentiating malignancy from acute benign compression fractures of the spine. AJNR Am J Neuroradiol 2006;27(6):1183–8.

[27] Baur A, Stabler A, Bruning R, et al. Diffusion-weighted MR imaging of bone marrow: differentiation of benign versus pathologic compression fractures. Radiology 1998;207(2): 349–56.

[28] Spuentrup E, Buecker A, Adam G, et al. Diffusion-weighted MR imaging for differentiation of benign fracture edema and tumor infiltration of the vertebral body. Am J Roentgenol 2001; 176(2):351–8.

[29] Baur A, Dietrich O, Reiser M. Diffusion-weighted imaging of bone marrow: current status. Eur Radiol 2003;13(7):1699–708.

[30] Saifuddin A, Bann K, Ridgaway JP, et al. Bone marrow blood supply in gadolinium-enhanced magnetic resonance imaging. Skeletal Radiol 1994;23(6):455–7.

[31] Griffith JF, Yeung DK, Antonio GE, et al. Vertebral bone mineral density, marrow perfusion, and fat content in healthy men and men with osteoporosis: dynamic contrast-enhanced MR imaging and MR spectroscopy. Radiology 2005; 236(3):945–51.

[32] Montazel JL, Divine M, Lepage E, et al. Normal spinal bone marrow in adults: dynamic gadolinium-enhanced MR imaging. Radiology 2003; 229(3):703–9.

[33] Sze G, Bravo S, Baierl P, et al. Developing spinal column: gadolinium-enhanced MR imaging. Radiology 1991;180(2):497–502.

[34] Rahmouni A, Montazel JL, Divine M, et al. Bone marrow with diffuse tumor infiltration in patients with lymphoproliferative diseases: dynamic gadolinium-enhanced MR imaging. Radiology 2003;229(3):710–7.

[35] Daldrup-Link HE, Rummeny EJ, Ihssen B, et al. Iron-oxide-enhanced MR imaging of bone marrow in patients with non-Hodgkin's lymphoma: differentiation between tumor infiltration and hypercellular bone marrow. Eur Radiol 2002;12(6):1557–66.

[36] Vande Berg BC, Lecouvet FE, Galant C, et al. Normal variants and frequent marrow alterations that simulate bone marrow lesions at MR imaging. Radiol Clin North Am 2005; 43(4):761–70.

[37] Ishijima H, Ishizaka H, Horikoshi H, et al. Water fraction of lumbar vertebral bone marrow estimated from chemical shift misregistration on MR imaging: normal variations with age and sex. Am J Roentgenol 1996;167(2): 355–8.

[38] Dunnill MS, Anderson JA, Whitehead R. Quantitative histological studies on age changes in bone. J Pathol Bacteriol 1967;94(2): 275–91.

[39] Schellinger D, Lin CS, Hatipoglu HG, et al. Potential value of vertebral proton MR spectroscopy in determining bone weakness. Am J Neuroradiol 2001;22(8):1620–7.

[40] Justesen J, Stenderup K, Ebbesen EN, et al. Adipocyte tissue volume in bone marrow is increased with aging and in patients with osteoporosis. Biogerontology 2001;2(3):165–71.

[41] Ricci C, Cova M, Kang YS, et al. Normal age-related patterns of cellular and fatty bone marrow distribution in the axial skeleton: MR imaging study. Radiology 1990;177(1): 83–8.

[42] Modic MT, Masaryk TJ, Ross JS, et al. Imaging of degenerative disk disease. Radiology 1988; 168(1):177–86.

[43] Hajek PC, Baker LL, Goobar JE, et al. Focal fat deposition in axial bone marrow: MR characteristics. Radiology 1987;162(1 Pt 1):245–9.

[44] Schweitzer ME, Levine C, Mitchell DG, et al. Bull's-eyes and halos: useful MR discriminators of osseous metastases. Radiology 1993;188(1): 249–52.

[45] Levine CD, Schweitzer ME, Ehrlich SM. Pelvic marrow in adults. Skeletal Radiol 1994;23(5): 343–7.

[46] Bordalo-Rodrigues M, Galant C, Lonneux M, et al. Focal nodular hyperplasia of the hematopoietic marrow simulating vertebral metastasis on FDG positron emission tomography. Am J Roentgenol 2003;180(3):669–71.

[47] Deutsch AL, Mink JH, Rosenfelt FP, et al. Incidental detection of hematopoietic hyperplasia on routine knee MR imaging. Am J Roentgenol 1989;152(2):333–6.

[48] Stabler A, Doma AB, Baur A, et al. Reactive bone marrow changes in infectious spondylitis: quantitative assessment with MR imaging. Radiology 2000;217(3):863–8.

[49] Fletcher BD, Wall JE, Hanna SL. Effect of hematopoietic growth factors on MR images of bone marrow in children undergoing chemotherapy. Radiology 1993;189(3):745–51.

[50] Durie BG, Kyle RA, Belch A, et al. Scientific advisors of the International Myeloma Foundation. Myeloma management guidelines: a consensus report from the scientific advisors of the International Myeloma Foundation. Hematol J 2003;4(6):379–98.

[51] Kyle RA, Therneau TM, Rajkumar SV, et al. A long term study of prognosis in monoclonal gammopathy of undetermined significance. N Engl J Med 2002;346:564–9.

[52] Bellaiche L, Laredo JD, Liote F, et al. Magnetic resonance appearance of monoclonal gammopathies of unknown significance and multiple myeloma. Spine 1997;22:2551–7.

[53] Mariette X, Zagdanski AM, Guermazi A, et al. Prognostic value of vertebral lesions detected by magnetic resonance imaging in patients with stage I multiple myeloma. Br J Haematol 1999;104(4):723–9.

[54] Vande Berg BC, Lecouvet FE, Michaux L, et al. Stage I multiple myeloma: value of MR imaging of the bone marrow in the determination of prognosis. Radiology 1996;201(1):243–6.

[55] Baur-Melnyk A, Buhmann S, Durr HR, et al. Role of MRI for the diagnosis and prognosis

[56] Lecouvet FE, Vande Berg BC, Michaux L, et al. Stage III multiple myeloma: clinical and prognostic value of spinal bone marrow MR imaging. Radiology 1998;209(3):653–60.

of multiple myeloma. Eur J Radiol 2005;55(1): 56–63.

[57] Stabler A, Baur A, Bartl R, et al. Contrast enhancement and quantitative signal analysis in MR imaging of multiple myeloma: assessment of focal and diffuse growth patterns in marrow correlated with biopsies and survival rates. Am J Roentgenol 1996;167(4):1029–36.

[58] Rahmouni A, Divine M, Mathieu D, et al. Detection of multiple myeloma involving the spine: efficacy of fat-suppression and contrast-enhanced MR imaging. Am J Roentgenol 1993; 160(5):1049–52.

[59] Baur A, Stabler A, Bartl R, et al. MRI gadolinium enhancement of bone marrow: age-related changes in normals and in diffuse neoplastic infiltration. Skeletal Radiol 1997;26(7):414–8.

[60] Moulopoulos LA, Dimopoulos MA. Magnetic resonance imaging of the bone marrow in hematologic malignancies. Blood 1997;90(6): 2127–47.

[61] Baur A, Bartl R, Pellengahr C, et al. Neovascularization of bone marrow in patients with diffuse multiple myeloma: a correlative study of magnetic resonance imaging and histopathologic findings. Cancer 2004;101(11):2599–604.

[62] Libshitz HI, Malthouse SR, Cunningham D, et al. Multiple myeloma: appearance at MR imaging. Radiology 1992;182(3):833–7.

[63] Moulopoulos LA, Dimopoulos MA, Smith TL, et al. Prognostic significance of magnetic resonance imaging in patients with asymptomatic multiple myeloma. J Clin Oncol 1995;13(1): 251–6.

[64] Baur A, Stabler A, Nagel D, et al. Magnetic resonance imaging as a supplement for the clinical staging system of Durie and Salmon? Cancer 2002;95(6):1334–45.

[65] Moulopoulos LA, Dimopoulos MA, Alexanian R, et al. Multiple myeloma: MR patterns of response to treatment. Radiology 1994;193(2):441–6.

[66] Duhem, Ries F, Dicato M. Accuracy of magnetic resonance imaging (MRI) of bone marrow in Waldenstrom's macroglobulinemia. Blood 1994; 84:653.

[67] Moulopoulos LA, Dimopoulos MA, Varma DGK, et al. Waldenstrom macroglobulinemia: MR imaging of the spine and CT of the abdomen and pelvis. Radiology 1993; 188(3):669–73.

[68] Gean-Marton AD, Kirsch CF, Vezina LG, et al. Focal amyloidosis of the head and neck: evaluation with CT and MR imaging. Radiology 1991;181(2):521–5.

[69] Ito M, Abumi K, Takeda N, et al. Pathologic features of spinal disorders in patients treated with long-term hemodialysis. Spine 1998;23(19): 2127–33.

[70] Campistol JM, Skinner M. Beta-2 microglobulin amyloidosis: an overview. Semin Dial 1993;6: 117–26.

[71] Faure C, Venin B, Bousquet JC, et al. Primary amyloidosis of bones. MRI aspects. J Radiol 1995;76(11):1025–7.

[72] Olliff JF, Hardy JR, Williams MP, et al. Magnetic resonance imaging of spinal amyloid. Clin Radiol 1989;40(6):632–3.

[73] Jensen KE, Sorensen PG, Thomsen C, et al. Prolonged T1 relaxation of the hemopoietic bone marrow in patients with chronic leukemia. Acta Radiol 1990;31(5):445–8.

[74] Lecouvet FE, Vande Berg BC, Michaux L, et al. Early chronic lymphocytic leukemia: prognostic value of quantitative bone marrow MR imaging findings and correlation with hematologic variables. Radiology 1997;204(3):813–8.

[75] Lecouvet FE, Vande Berg BC, Michaux L, et al. Chronic lymphocytic leukemia: changes in bone marrow composition and distribution assessed with quantitative MRI. J Magn Reson Imaging 1998;8(3):733–9.

[76] Bongers H, Schick F, Skalej M, et al. Localized in vivo 1H spectroscopy and chemical shift imaging of the bone marrow in leukemic patients. Eur Radiol 1992;4(2):350–6.

[77] Gerard EL, Ferry JA, Amrein PC, et al. Compositional changes in vertebral bone marrow during treatment for acute leukemia: assessment with quantitative chemical shift imaging. Radiology 1992;183(1):39–46.

[78] Schick F, Einsele H, Lutz O, et al. Lipid selective MR imaging and localized 1H spectroscopy of bone marrow during therapy of leukemia. Anticancer Res 1996;16(3B):1545–51.

[79] Vande Berg BC, Schmitz PJ, Scheiff JM, et al. Acute myeloid leukemia: lack of predictive value of sequential quantitative MR imaging during treatment. Radiology 1995;197(1):301–5.

[80] Jensen KE, Grundtvig Sorensen P, Thomsen C, et al. Magnetic resonance imaging of the bone marrow in patients with acute leukemia during and after chemotherapy. Changes in T1 relaxation. Acta Radiol 1990;31(4):361–9.

[81] Vande Berg BC, Michaux L, Scheiff JM, et al. Sequential quantitative MR analysis of bone marrow: differences during treatment of lymphoid versus myeloid leukemia. Radiology 1996; 201(2):519–23.

[82] Pui MH, Fletcher BD, Langston JW. Granulocytic sarcoma in childhood leukemia: imaging features. Radiology 1994;190(3):698–702.

[83] Moulopoulos LA, Maris TG, Papanikolaou N, et al. Detection of malignant bone marrow involvement with dynamic contrast-enhanced magnetic resonance imaging. Ann Oncol 2003; 14(1):152–8.

[84] Kaplan KR, Mitchell DG, Steiner RM, et al. Polycythemia vera and myelofibrosis: correlation of MR imaging, clinical, and laboratory findings. Radiology 1992;183(2):329–34.

[85] Padhani A, Husband J. Bone. In: Husband JES, Reznek RH, editors. Imaging in oncology. Oxford (UK): Isis Medical Media; 1998. p. 765–86.

[86] Algra PR, Bloem JL, Tissing H, et al. Detection of vertebral metastases: comparison between MR imaging and bone scintigraphy. Radiographics 1991;11(2):219–32.

[87] Colman LK, Porter BA, Redmond J 3rd, et al. Early diagnosis of spinal metastases by CT and MR studies. J Comput Assist Tomogr 1988; 12(3):423–6.

[88] Kattapuram SV, Khurana JS, Scott JA, et al. Negative scintigraphy with positive magnetic resonance imaging in bone metastases. Skeletal Radiol 1990;19(2):113–6.

[89] Kim HJ, Ryu KN, Choi WS, et al. Spinal involvement of hematopoietic malignancies and metastasis: differentiation using MR imaging. Clin Imaging 1999;23(2):125–33.

[90] Baker LL, Goodman SB, Perkash I, et al. Benign versus pathologic compression fractures of vertebral bodies: assessment with conventional spin-echo, chemical shift, and STIR MR imaging. Radiology 1990;174(2):495–502.

[91] Resnick D, Niwayama G. Osteoporosis. In: Resnick D, editor. Diagnosis of bone and joint disorders. 3rd edition. Philadephia: WB Saunders; 1995. p. 1837–9.

[92] Yuh WT, Zachar CK, Barloon TJ, et al. Vertebral compression fractures: distinction between benign and malignant causes with MR imaging. Radiology 1989;172(1):215–8.

[93] Baur A, Stabler A, Arbogast S, et al. Acute osteoporotic and neoplastic vertebral compression fractures: fluid sign at MR imaging. Radiology 2002;225(3):730–8.

[94] Lo LD, Schweitzer ME, Juneja V, et al. Are L5 fractures an indicator of metastasis? Skeletal Radiol 2000;29(8):454–8.

[95] Baur A, Huber A, Ertl-Wagner B, et al. Diagnostic value of increased diffusion weighting of a steady-state free precession sequence for differentiating acute benign osteoporotic fractures from pathologic vertebral compression fractures. Am J Neuroradiol 2001;22(2): 366–72.

[96] Baur A, Huber A, Durr HR, et al. Differentiation of benign osteoporotic and neoplastic vertebral compression fractures with a diffusion-weighted, steady-state free precession sequence. Rofo 2002;174(1):70–5.

[97] Pond GD, Castellino RA, Horning S, et al. Non-Hodgkin lymphoma: influence of lymphography, CT, and bone marrow biopsy on staging and management. Radiology 1989;170(1 Pt 1): 159–64.

[98] Howell SJ, Grey M, Chang J, et al. The value of bone marrow examination in the staging of Hodgkin's lymphoma: a review of 955 cases seen in a regional cancer centre. Br J Haematol 2002;119(2):408–11.

[99] Linden A, Zankovich R, Theissen P, et al. Malignant lymphoma: bone marrow imaging versus biopsy. Radiology 1989;173(2):335–9.

[100] Vourtsi AD, Moulopoulos LA, Gouliamos A, et al. The "wrap-around" MR sign: a telltale sign of lymphoma of the bone marrow. Eur Radiol 1997;7:S390.

[101] Varan A, Cila A, Buyukpamukcu M. Prognostic importance of magnetic resonance imaging in bone marrow involvement of Hodgkin disease. Med Pediatr Oncol 1999;32(4):267–71.

[102] Tardivon AA, Munck JN, Shapeero LG, et al. Can clinical data help to screen patients with lymphoma for MR imaging of bone marrow? Ann Oncol 1995;6(8):795–800.

[103] Smith R, Schilder K, Shaer A, et al. Lymphoma staging with bone marrow MRI. Proc Am Soc Clin Oncol 1995;14:390.

[104] Kusumoto S, Jinnai I, Matsuda A, et al. Bone marrow patterns in patients with aplastic anaemia and myelodysplastic syndrome: observations with magnetic resonance imaging. Eur J Haematol 1997;59(3):155–61.

[105] Katsuya T, Inoue T, Ishizaka H, et al. Dynamic contrast-enhanced MR imaging of the water fraction of normal bone marrow and diffuse bone marrow disease. Radiat Med 2000;18(5): 291–7.

[106] Negendank W, Weissman D, Bey TM, et al. Evidence for clonal disease by magnetic resonance imaging in patients with hypoplastic marrow disorders. Blood 1991;78(11):2872–9.

[107] Bayik M, Kodalli N, Gürmen N, et al. Magnetic resonance imaging in myelofibrosis. Blood 1998; 92(8):2995–7.

[108] Roca M, Mota J, Giraldo P, et al. Systemic mastocytosis: MRI of bone marrow involvement. Eur Radiol 1999;9(6):1094–7.

[109] Hauswirth AW, Simonitsch-Klupp I, Uffmann M, et al. Response to therapy with interferon alpha-2b and prednisolone in aggressive systemic mastocytosis: report of five cases and review of the literature. Leuk Res 2004;28(3):249–57.

[110] Avila NA, Ling A, Metcalfe DD, et al. Mastocytosis: magnetic resonance imaging patterns of marrow disease. Skeletal Radiol 1998;27(3): 119–26.

[111] Resnick D, Haghighi P. Myeloproliferative disorders. In: Resnick D, editor. Diagnosis of bone and joint disorders. 3rd edition. (vol. 4). Philadelphia: WB Saunders; 1995. p. 2483–7.

[112] Ho LM, Lipper MH. Mastocytosis of the axial skeleton presenting as an epidural mass lesion: MR imaging appearance. Am J Roentgenol 1996;167(3):716–8.

[113] Haney K, Russell W, Raila FA, et al. MRI characteristics of systemic mastocytosis of the lumbosacral spine. Skeletal Radiol 1996;25(2):171–3.

[114] Levin TL, Sheth SS, Hurlet A, et al. MR marrow signs of iron overload in transfusion-dependent patients with sickle cell disease. Pediatr Radiol 1995;25(8):614–9.

[115] Charrow J, Esplin JA, Gribble TJ, et al. Gaucher disease: recommendations on diagnosis, evaluation, and monitoring. Arch Intern Med 1998; 158(16):1754–60.

[116] Rosenthal DI, Scott JA, Barranger J, et al. Evaluation of Gaucher disease using magnetic resonance imaging. J Bone Joint Surg Am 1986; 68(6):802–8.

[117] Hermann G, Shapiro RS, Fikry Abdelwahab I, et al. MR imaging in adults with Gaucher disease type 1: evaluation of marrow involvement and disease activity. Skeletal Radiol 1993;22(4):247–51.

[118] Maas M, van Kuijk C, Stoker J, et al. Quantification of bone involvement in Gaucher disease: MR imaging bone marrow burden score as an alternative to Dixon quantitative chemical shift MR imaging-initial experience. Radiology 2003; 229(2):554–61.

[119] Stevens SK, Moore SG, Kaplan ID. Early and late bone-marrow changes after irradiation: MR evaluation. Am J Roentgenol 1990;154(4):745–50.

[120] Mitchell MJ, Logan PM. Radiation-induced changes in bone. Radiographics 1998;18(5): 1125–36.

[121] Yankelevitz DF, Henschke CI, Knapp PH, et al. Effect of radiation therapy on thoracic and lumbar bone marrow: evaluation with MR imaging. Am J Roentgenol 1991;157(1):87–92.

[122] Otake S, Mayr NA, Ueda T, et al. Radiation-induced changes in MR signal intensity and contrast enhancement of lumbosacral vertebrae: do changes occur only inside the radiation therapy field? Radiology 2002;222(1):179–83.

[123] Sacks EL, Goris ML, Glatstein E, et al. Bone marrow regeneration following large field radiation. Cancer 1978;42(3):1057–65.

[124] Lieschke GJ, Burgess AW. Granulocyte colony-stimulating factor and granulocyte-macrophage colony-stimulating factor. N Engl J Med 1992; 327(1):28–35.

[125] Ciray I, Lindman H, Astrom GK, et al. Effect of granulocyte colony-stimulating factor (G-CSF)-supported chemotherapy on MR imaging of normal red bone marrow in breast cancer patients with focal bone metastases. Acta Radiol 2003;44(5):472–84.

[126] Hartman RP, Sundaram M, Okuno SH, et al. Effect of granulocyte-stimulating factors on marrow of adult patients with musculoskeletal malignancies: incidence and MRI findings. Am J Roentgenol 2004;183(3): 645–53.

[127] Altehoefer C, Bertz H, Ghanem NA, et al. Extent and time course of morphological changes of bone marrow induced by granulocyte-colony stimulating factor as assessed by magnetic resonance imaging of healthy blood stem cell donors. J Magn Reson Imaging 2001;14(2): 141–6.

[128] Stevens SK, Moore SG, Amylon MD. Repopulation of the marrow after transplantation: MR imaging with pathologic correlation. Radiology 1990;175(1):213–8.

[129] Tanner SF, Clarke J, Leach MO, et al. MRI in the evaluation of late bone marrow changes following bone marrow transplantation. Br J Radiol 1996;69(828):1145–51.

[130] Pereira PL, Schick F, Einsele H, et al. MR tomography of the bone marrow changes after high-dosage chemotherapy and autologous peripheral stem-cell transplantation. Rofo 1999; 170(3):251–7.

MAGNETIC
RESONANCE
IMAGING CLINICS

Magn Reson Imaging Clin N Am 15 (2007) 221–238

ELSEVIER
SAUNDERS

Imaging the Degenerative Diseases of the Lumbar Spine

David Malfair, MD[a], Douglas P. Beall, MD[b,c],*

Degenerative diseases of the spine are a ubiquitous collection of conditions that represent some of the most common indications for advanced imaging studies. Degenerative change of the nucleus pulposis is termed intervertebral osteochondrosis. Altered biomechanics may occur secondary to intervertebral osteochondrosis and may contribute to the progression to annular tears, disc herniations, degenerative end plate changes, and Schmorl's nodes. Spondylosis deformans represents an additional degenerative process of the disc. It is characterized by osteophytes that occur at attachment sites of the perivertebral ligaments of the outer annulus fibrosis to the vertebral periosteum. The diarthrodial facet joints are frequently affected by degenerative osteoarthrosis in a manner similar to other synovial articulations throughout the body. Degenerative changes in the ligamentum flavum, the interspinous ligaments, and the posterior longitudinal ligament are also frequently detected on cross-sectional imaging studies. Familiarity with the normal anatomy and the manifestations of degenerative changes of these structures is necessary for optimal diagnosis.

MR imaging is often the modality of choice in assessing degenerative changes within the spine because of its superior soft tissue contrast. CT demonstrates superior spatial resolution and provides improved conspicuity of osseous and calcified structures. CT, however, is less sensitive than MR imaging in detecting soft tissue degenerative changes because it relies on prominent alterations in the tissue planes before pathologic changes can be detected in the anatomy. Other imaging tests may be helpful, especially when the clinical presentation and MR imaging findings are discordant. Complementary tests in the evaluation of degenerative spinal disease include radiography, discography, conventional myelography, CT myelography, and nuclear scintigraphy.

[a] Division of Radiology, University of California San Francisco, 505 Parnassus Avenue, San Francisco, CA 94143-628, USA
[b] Clinical Radiology of Oklahoma, P.O. Box 721688, Oklahoma City, OK 73172-1688, USA
[c] University of Oklahoma, 610 NW 14th Street, Oklahoma City, OK 73103, USA
* Corresponding author. University of Oklahoma, 610 NW 14th Street, Oklahoma City, OK 73103.
E-mail address: dpb@okss.com (D.P. Beall).

1064-9689/07/$ – see front matter © 2007 Published by Elsevier Inc.   doi:10.1016/j.mric.2007.04.001
mri.theclinics.com

Degenerative change may present with local back pain, radiculopathy, or myelopathy. Degenerative facet arthropathy, degenerative disc disease, degenerative end plate changes, and ligamentous injury are all possible pain generators in the setting of axial back pain [1–3]. Narrowing of the spinal canal or neural foramina can result in myelopathy and radiculopathy, respectively. Segmental instability, kyphosis, and scoliosis are examples of malalignment that may occur secondary to degenerative disease. Imaging of patients who have suspected spine pathology characterizes the level and extent of degenerative changes that may be a source of symptoms. Significant morphologic changes on imaging are often found in asymptomatic patients [4–7], which underscores the need for a thorough clinical assessment and provides support for acquiring electrophysiologic data when necessary to determine the significance of anatomic findings seen on imaging studies.

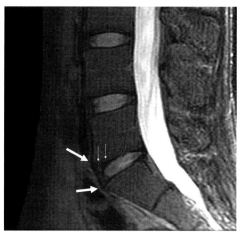

Fig. 1. Normal disc anatomy. T2-weighted sagittal MR image of the lumbar spine with fat saturation demonstrates homogenous high signal in the central nucleus pulposis (*black arrow*). The inner fibers of the annulus (*small white arrows*) attach directly to the end plate and the outer fibers (*large white arrows*) attach to the vertebral periosteum.

Degenerative disc changes in the anterior elements

Intervertebral osteochondrosis

The intervertebral disc space is a cartilaginous or amphiarthrodial joint with a central nucleus pulposis surrounded by an annulus fibrosis. The nucleus pulposis consists primarily of hydrated proteoglycans supported by an irregular network of elastin and fine collagen type II fibers. The annulus fibrosis is composed of an outer and inner layer. The outer layer consists mainly of collagen type 1 fibers and is anchored to the vertebral rim and vertebral periosteum by way of the perivertebral ligaments. The inner annulus fibrosis is composed of fibrocartilage and collagen and attaches to the cartilaginous end plate (Fig. 1). Together, they resist axial loading while allowing limited movements. The nucleus pulposis converts much of the axial force into a radial force and functions to spread the loading more evenly over the adjacent end plate.

Terminology regarding degenerative disc disease can be confusing. It has been suggested that the term "early degenerative changes" should refer to accelerated age-related changes in the disc without evidence of structural failure [3]. A degenerated disc is a term reserved for those with structural failure combined with accelerated or advanced signs of aging. Degenerative disc disease is best defined as symptomatic degenerative disc changes. Many patients exhibit degenerative changes without associated symptoms. Matsumoto and colleagues [4] noted that approximately 90% of asymptomatic patients over 60 years old demonstrate some cervical disc degeneration.

Degeneration of the nucleus pulposis is characterized by progressive desiccation and fragmentation of the glycosaminoglycan content [7]. Whether these biochemical changes cause, or are the result of, mechanical disc degeneration is subject to debate [8–11]. The adult nucleus pulposis has a limited blood supply and the nutrient vessels are restricted to the outermost layers of the annulus, with the remainder of the disc supplied by metabolite diffusion. This relative lack of blood supply and the sparse cell population within the nucleus results in limited ability to recover from metabolic or mechanical injury. Gross injuries to a disc may never fully heal [12]. As disc injury progresses, loss of intradiscal pressure may result in decreased disc height, annular tears, and disc herniation.

MR imaging is sensitive for early changes of intervertebral osteochondrosis. The classification proposed by Pffirman and colleagues [13] for the MR imaging features of internal disc degeneration is based on sagittal fast spin-echo T2-weighted sequences. Early disc changes on MR imaging include loss of normal homogenous T2 hyperintensity within the nucleus (Fig. 2). Later changes involve decreasing signal within the nucleus pulposis, with loss of the normal distinction between the nucleus pulposis and the annulus fibrosis. Progressive disc height loss and disc bulges characterize the later changes in more severely degenerated discs. Posterior osteophytes also can occur at this stage and may contribute to spinal and foraminal stenosis. Radial expansion and remodeling of the

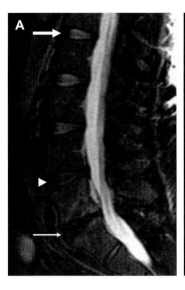
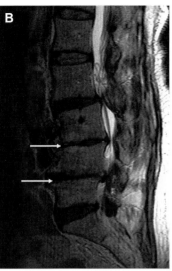

Fig. 2. Disc degeneration. (*A*) Sagittal short tau inversion recovery MR image shows discs with early degenerative changes (*thick white arrow*) that demonstrate a horizontal low intensity line, the intranuclear cleft. As discs further degenerate, the distinction between the nucleus pulposis and the annulus fibrosis becomes less distinct (*white arrowhead*). More prominently degenerated discs (*thin white arrow*) are completely hypointense. (*B*) T2-weighted sagittal midline MR image (with fat saturation) shows multiple levels of advanced degenerative disc changes including a uniformly low signal within the disc and decreased disc height (*thin white arrows*).

vertebral body with increase in the anteroposterior dimension can also occur (Fig. 3).

Conventional radiography and CT imaging are insensitive for detecting early degenerative disc changes. CT can be helpful in characterizing later changes, including detecting disc calcification and differentiating osteophyte from degenerated portions of the intervertebral disc [14,15]. Gas in the

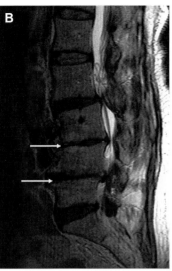

Fig. 3. Degenerative kyphosis. T1-weighted sagittal image of the thoracic spine demonstrates loss of anterior disc height (*arrows*) in the midthoracic spine, resulting in a thoracic kyphosis. Increased anteroposterior dimension of these vertebral bodies is likely secondary to chronic remodeling.

disc space is almost pathognomonic for disc degeneration, although it also may be seen occasionally in trauma and some infections [16]. Intervertebral disc height at the lumbosacral junction is variable because of segmentation differences and a decreased disc height at this interspace is not necessarily pathologic (Fig. 4).

Annular tears

Annular tears represent a biomechanical failure of the annulus fibrosis and are usually associated with degenerative changes in the nucleus pulposis [17,18]. The three basic types of annular tears are vertical, radial, and peripheral rim tears. Radial tears extend from the inner margin of the annulus to the periphery, and usually occur posteriorly or posterolaterally. Radial annular tears are important in that they are a precursor to disc herniation and a potential cause for axial back pain. Vertical and peripheral rim tearing of the intervertebral disc may also occur but is of uncertain clinical significance. Vertical tears or "delamination" occur secondary to laminar shear stress. These tears occur between the concentric fibers of the annulus fibrosis. Peripheral rim tears occur at the attachment of the outer fibers of the annulus fibrosis to the vertebral periosteum. They are more frequently seen anteriorly [18] and are associated with spondylosis deformans.

Annular tears may be optimally detected on the T1-weighted sequences after administration of gadolinium because this sequence may be the most sensitive for detecting annular tears [19,20]. Granulation tissue within the tear can demonstrate high signal on the T2-weighted sequences and is referred

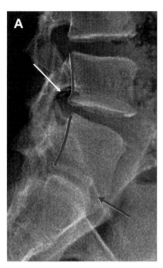 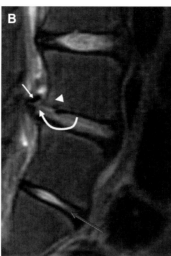

Fig. 4. Adolescent disc herniation. (*A*) Lateral conventional radiograph demonstrates disc height loss and retrolisthesis (posterior vertebral body walls at the affected level indicated by black lines). A small osseous fragment (*white arrow*) suggests the presence of an apophyseal ring disruption. (*B*) T2-weighted sagittal MR imaging sequence demonstrates posterior intervertebral disc herniation (*curved white arrow*) and T2 prolongation in the subchondral marrow at the donor site (*white arrowhead*). The small osseous fragment is also noted along the posterosuperior portion of the disc herniation (*small white arrow*). Also note the normal disc at the L5–S1 level despite narrow disc space (*black arrows in A and B*).

to as a high intensity zone (Fig. 5) [21,22]. These changes may persist for years on follow-up studies and therefore do not necessarily represent an acute or subacute event [23]. Severely degenerated discs with loss of T2 prolongation and disc height invariably demonstrate annular tears on provocative discography [24]. MR imaging demonstrates only moderate sensitivity in the detection of annular tears in cadaver studies [17,25], especially vertical tears which, are only occasionally detected on MR imaging. Sensitivity for the detection of radial tears may be increased with the application of an axial load [26].

Discography is also used to evaluate annular tears. It involves a percutaneous injection of contrast into the nucleus pulposis in an attempt to assess the integrity of the annulus fibrosis. Because the contrast is injected under high pressure, patients are asked to correlate the type, quality, and severity of back pain elicited. CT after discography improves the sensitivity for detecting small annular tears (see Fig. 3). CT discography is also more sensitive than MR in detecting radial annular tears [27]. Discography cannot detect concentric or peripheral rim tears because these tears do not communicate with the nucleus pulposis.

Annular tears are of uncertain clinical significance. Some investigators believe that these changes represent normal aging. Tears are noted frequently in asymptomatic patients [27] and in nearly all severely degenerated discs. Degeneration of the disc can cause marked axial back pain, and a significant

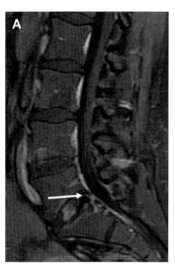 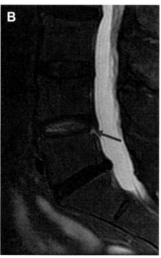

Fig. 5. Annular tear. (*A*) T1-weighted sagittal MR image with fat saturation obtained after an intravenous gadolinium injection demonstrates an enhancing annular tear or high intensity zone (*white arrow*). (*B*) T2-weighted sagittal image with fat saturation in a second patient demonstrates an extensive radial tear of the intervertebral disc extending to the posterior outer annular fibers (*black arrow*). Increased intradiscal signal on the T2-weighted images occurs secondary to granulation tissue within the tear. This increased signal was unchanged on a 6-month follow-up examination (not shown).

number of patients obtain relief with discectomy and fusion or total lumbar disc replacement [19]. Despite this, surgery for axial back pain is often unsuccessful and selecting those patients whose axial back pain will improve after intervertebral disc surgery is challenging. Numerous studies have promoted discography as a means of confirming that a disc is a pain generator in patients who have otherwise unexplained axial back pain [19,28]. The diagnosis of discogenic back pain, however, is very difficult and discography is an imperfect gold standard. Reported false-positive rates are high in asymptomatic patients, ranging from 20% to 40% [29,30]. Despite careful selection of patients with discography, the success rate of surgery for discogenic back pain ranges from 40% to 60% [30,31].

Disc herniation

Nomenclature regarding disc herniation varies widely and is often confusing. Standardized definitions have been introduced by the North American Spine Society [32]. According to these definitions, a herniation is defined as a localized displacement of disc material beyond the limits of the periphery of the disc. Several modifiers were described to standardize spinal nomenclature further. A herniation is "focal" if it involves less than 25% of the disc circumference. A "broad-based" disc herniation involves between 25% and 50% of the disc circumference, and involvement of more than 50% of the circumference of the disc is defined as a "disc bulge." A "disc protrusion" is defined as a herniation that demonstrates broad continuity with the adjacent disc. If the size of the disc fragment (in any plane) is greater than the width of the base, it is termed a "disc extrusion" (Fig. 6). A "sequestered disc"

refers to a disc fragment that has lost all continuity with the parent disc.

Disc herniations are also described by their position. In the axial plane, they may be central, subarticular (paracentral), foraminal, or extraforaminal in location (Fig. 7). Ninety percent of disc herniations are central or paracentral in location. Five percent are noted in the foramen and 5% are extraforaminal. Most disc herniations occur in the lumbar spine. The cervical spine is the next most common region that is affected by intervertebral disc herniation. Thoracic disc herniations are the least common, but may be underrecognized. Disc herniation may cause narrowing of the spinal canal and neural foramina. Compression of neural structures should be described in terms of location and severity.

MR imaging is an excellent modality for characterizing disc herniations, and demonstrates a high specificity and sensitivity. The excellent soft tissue contrast of MR imaging allows depiction of nerve roots and the spinal cord within the thecal sac. Encroachment on these structures from soft tissue and osseous structures is easily recognized. Disc extrusions and protrusions are continuous with the disc and are usually of similar signal to disc on all sequences [33]. The degree of T2 prolongation varies with the extent of disc degeneration [34]. When the discs are of very low signal on T2 sequences, MR may not allow a distinction between the relative contributions of osseous and soft tissue elements to the degree of stenosis that is present [35]. This situation commonly occurs in the cervical spine where distinction between a hard bony narrowing and soft disc narrowing may affect treatment options [36]. CT can be a complementary modality in this circumstance because it easily

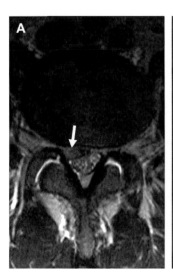 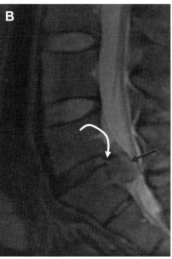

Fig. 6. Disc herniation. (*A*) T2-weighted axial MR image with fat saturation shows a broad-based right central/subarticular disc protrusion (*white arrow*). (*B*) T2-weighted sagittal MR image with fat saturation demonstrates a large central extrusion (*black arrow*) with narrow connection to the disc of origin (*curved white arrow*).

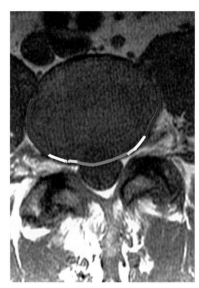

Fig. 7. Axial T1-weighted MR image of the lumbar spine shows the zones of intervertebral disc herniation (green zone: central zone; yellow zone: subarticular zone; white zone: foraminal zone; red zone: extraforaminal zone).

of a fragment suggests a larger annular defect and has been associated with higher rates of recurrence [41]. The presence of a minimally degenerated disc has also been shown to be associated with greater rates of recurrent disc herniation after surgery. Dora and colleagues [42] observed that patients who had minimal MR evidence of disc degeneration had a 6.8 fold relative risk of symptomatic recurrent disc herniation after surgery relative to those patients who had marked disc degeneration.

Herniation in adolescents is an important topic because it has unique pathologic and imaging features. Herniation is often associated with concomitant disruption of the posterior apophyseal ring, which can be observed on lateral conventional radiographs, CT scans, and MR imaging [43,44] (see Fig. 6; Fig. 9). MR imaging delineates the size of the herniated fragment and the presence and location of a displaced osseous fragment such as a portion of the apophyseal ring (see Fig. 4). This avulsed fragment can ossify and result in spinal stenosis. Disagreement exists as to whether the identification of apophyseal ring disruption is an indication for surgery [45,46].

Degenerative end plate changes

End plate changes adjacent to disc degeneration are common and are best characterized on MR imaging [47,48]. Degenerative end plate changes are identified in 20% to 50% of patients and may be classified according to their signal abnormalities on MR imaging. The typical classification system used to categorize the degenerative end plate changes is the Modic classification system developed by Michael Modic in the late 1980s. Type I Modic degenerative endplate changes consist of decreased signal

demonstrates the posterior osteophyte component of a disc/osteophyte complex that can cause spinal canal or neural foraminal narrowing. CT may also be useful in cases where MR and clinical findings are not congruent and surgery is being considered.

Sequestered disc fragments may be challenging to identify on MR imaging. They are of variable signal intensity on T1- and T2-weighted sequences, but contrast-enhanced studies can aid in their identification and characterization. These disc fragments commonly demonstrate peripheral enhancement on the postgadolinium administration sequences (Fig. 8). Sequestered discs are most often found just anterior to the posterior longitudinal ligament in the anterior epidural space. Dorsal displacement of the posterior longitudinal ligament can be a clue to their location.

The presence of disc herniation does not correlate well with symptoms and does not predict future symptoms [5,37,38]. Chung and colleagues [39] described the prevalence rate of disc protrusion as 20% in patients without a history of back pain. Weishaupt and colleagues [5] found disc bulges and protrusions in most of the asymptomatic volunteers that they examined with MR imaging. Most disc extrusions are symptomatic but this more severe type of disc herniation may also be found in asymptomatic patients.

A recurrent disc herniation is a common reason for an unsatisfactory outcome after surgery and occurs with a prevalence of 5% to 20% [40]. Extrusion

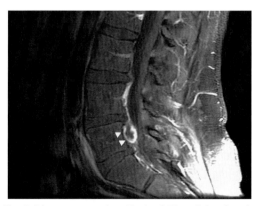

Fig. 8. Disc sequestration. Sagittal T1-weighted sagittal image with gadolinium demonstrates peripheral enhancement of a sequestered disc (*arrowheads*) in the anterior epidural space between the L5 vertebral body and the posterior longitudinal ligament.

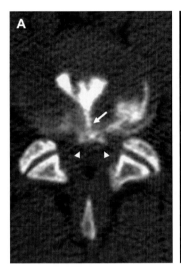
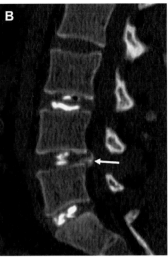

Fig. 9. CT discogram. (*A*) Axial CT image obtained after conventional discography shows a central annular tear (*white arrow*) with contrast extending into a small central disc protrusion (*white arrowheads*). (*B*) Sagittal reformatted CT image performed after conventional discography demonstrates a posterior central full-thickness radial annular tear (*white arrow*).

intensity on the T1-weighted images and increased signal intensity on the T2-weighted images. Histologic examination shows increased vascularity within the subchondral bone along with fissuring of the cartilaginous end plates. Type II Modic degenerative end plate changes follow fat on all MR sequences (Fig. 10). Fatty replacement is visualized in samples taken from vertebral bodies with Modic type 2 degenerative end plate changes. This histology is thought to represent the sequelae of chronic marrow ischemia [49]. Type III Modic changes are characterized by regions of decreased signal on all MR sequences. This decreased signal represents end plate sclerosis. Type I Modic changes rarely regress and most commonly progress to type II changes. Over time, type 1 and 2 degenerative end plate changes may occasionally progress to type III changes.

Type 1 Modic degenerative end plate change has been positively correlated with the presence of back pain [48–52]. Degenerative end plate changes, however, are also found in 10% to 25% of asymptomatic volunteers [5,39]. Chung and colleagues [39] noted that asymptomatic degenerative end plate changes were different in distribution and morphology, compared with those of symptomatic patients examined by Modic and colleagues [48]. The asymptomatic changes were generally focal, located in the anterosuperior end plate, and centered in the midlumbar spine. The adjacent disc was

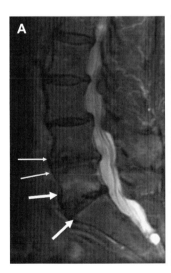
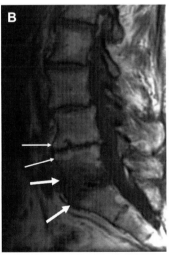

Fig. 10. Degenerative end plate changes. (*A*) Sagittal T2-weighted MR image with fat saturation shows primarily Modic type 2 degenerative end plate changes at the L4–5 level (*thin white arrows*) that follows fat tissue. Increased T2 signal is seen just subjacent to the inferior end plate of L5 and similar, but more subtle, changes in the superior portion of S1 (*thick white arrows*), consistent with Modic type 1 changes. (*B*) Sagittal T1-weighted MR image shows fat signal immediately adjacent to the L4–5 intervertebral level (*thin white arrows*), consistent with Modic type 2 degenerative end plate changes. The image also shows decreased signal in the inferior portion of the L5 vertebral body and the superior-most portion of the S1 vertebral body, consistent with Modic type 1 degenerative end plate change (*thick white arrows*).

usually unremarkable. The degenerative end plate changes in symptomatic patients studied by Modic and colleagues typically demonstrated confluent end plate changes superior and inferior to a degenerated disc. These changes were usually found in the lower lumbar spine.

Schmorl's nodes represent herniations of the nucleus pulposis into the subchondral bone through the associated vertebral end plate, a frequent finding in patients with a reported prevalence on MR imaging studies ranging from 9% to 38% [53]. Most of these nodes occur in the middle and posterior thirds of the end plate and between the levels of T7 and L2. In most cases, they represent remote occurrences and are of no clinical consequence.

Most intraosseous end plate herniations occur after axial loading and result in preferential extrusion of nuclear material through the vertebral end plate rather than through an intact annulus fibrosis. The annulus fibrosis is biomechically stronger than the end plate in young individuals. Intrinsic abnormalities of the end plate caused by vascular channels or small defects from notochordal remnants result in additional predisposition to end plate herniations [54]. Schmorl's nodes are also found more frequently in patients lacking a concave contour of the end plate [53]. A straight end plate demonstrates a less favorable biomechanical distribution of axial loading and end plate herniations may be found either in the setting of acute trauma or as an incidental finding noted on an imaging study acquired for reasons other than back pain. Acute Schmorl's nodes with associated fracture and hemorrhage were noted in 10% of patients in an autopsy study of motor vehicle collisions [55]. Schmorl's nodes in this setting can certainly be a source of axial back pain [56,57].

Schmorl's nodes are visualized well on both CT and MR imaging [56,58]. On CT, a focal indentation in the end plate is seen to communicate with the associated intervertebral disc. The Schmorl's node may also have bony sclerosis surrounding the portion of the disc that herniates into the vertebral body. MR imaging demonstrates direct continuity of the disc into the material that has herniated through the end plate. MR imaging may also demonstrate increased T2 signal in the adjacent bone marrow, a finding that has been found more commonly in patients who have symptomatic back pain and may represent an acute/subacute Schmorl's node [57]. In this setting, the areas of high T2 signal in the marrow typically follow the contour of the end plate (Fig. 11). Postcontrast T1-weighted sequences obtained after intravenous administration of gadolinium may also demonstrate enhancement of the herniated nucleus pulposis [56].

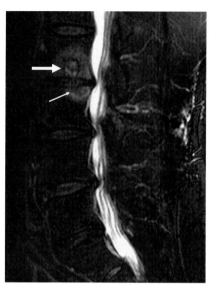

Fig. 11. Acute Schmorl's node. T2-weighted sagittal MR image with fat saturation demonstrates an end plate herniation through the inferior end plate of L2 (*large white arrow*) and edema resulting from the end plate herniation through the superior end plate of L3 (*small white arrow*).

Spondylosis deformans

Spondylosis deformans is an entity distinct from osteoarthritis and spondylitis. The primary finding in spondylosis deformans is the presence of osteophytes, which occur secondary to chronic traction stress at attachment sites of the Sharpey's fibers. The Sharpey's fibers from the annulus fibrosis attach to the vertebral periosteum and to the anterior longitudinal ligament. Osteophytes are found in most patients over 50 years old and usually occur 2 to 3 mm from the discovertebral junction, at the site of the Sharpey's fibers attachment. These have an initial horizontal orientation, which helps distinguish them from syndesmophytes (which are typically vertically oriented and found in seronegative arthropathies) [51]. Anterior osteophytes are very common and are usually asymptomatic.

Degenerative change of the uncovertebral joints

Uncovertebral joints are found from the C2–3 to the C6–7 level of the cervical spine. They are not present in the infant, but develop between the uncinate process of the lower vertebrae and the lateral margin of the more superior vertebrae [51]. These joints are lined with cartilage that is continuous and presumably originates from the adjacent cartilaginous end plate. These joints are variable and are not found in all individuals at all levels.

The primary clinical importance of the uncovertebral joint is its role in neural foraminal narrowing and resultant nerve root compromise. Because disc degeneration results in disc height loss of the cervical spine, the uncovertebral articulations are pressed firmly together. The joints then undergo degeneration, resulting in osteophytes that typically narrow the neural foramina [59]. Neural foraminal narrowing may result in nerve root compromise that produces radiculopathy, but uncovertebral joint degenerative change without radiculopathy is also seen very commonly [6].

Degenerative changes in the posterior elements

Degenerative changes of the facet joints

Osteoarthritis of the facet joints is thought to be secondary to repeated stress and trauma with secondary overload. The inciting event is thought to be fibrillation and erosion of articular cartilage, which progresses to joint space narrowing, sclerosis, and osteophyte formation. Abnormal stresses across the facet joint can also result in hypertrophy of the articular process, a distinct entity from osteophyte formation [60]. Facet degenerative changes are most commonly found in the mid- to lower cervical spine and the lower lumbar spine. Patients usually present with findings of axial pain but may also present with signs of radiculopathy or myelopathy.

Many investigators favor the hypothesis that disc degeneration precedes, and is one of the main inciting factors for, facet osteoarthrosis [61–63]. Facet arthropathy is much more commonly seen in the presence of marked disc degeneration, and disc degeneration most often anatomically precedes the development of facet arthropathy [61]. Narrowing of the disc results in cranial subluxation of the superior articular process (of the vertebral level below the disc) relative to the inferior articular process (of the vertebral level above the disc) and alters the stress on the facet joint itself [62]. Biomechanical studies demonstrate increased loading on facets, with narrowing of the disc space [63]. Increased mobility at a segment, often seen in early disc degeneration, can also contribute to facet arthropathy [62]. Facet tropism (asymmetry) and the more sagittal orientation of the facet joints are other hypothesized causes for facet degeneration [64]. Whether these associations are causative factors or the result of osseous remodeling to abnormal stresses is unknown.

Degenerative facet arthropathy is seen to some degree in most individuals over 50 years old and is frequently asymptomatic. However, pain originating from facet joints with relief after therapeutic injection, nerve ablation, or surgery is well documented [65–67]. The typical findings of facet joint arthropathy seen on CT include osteophyte formation, subchondral sclerosis, cyst formation, and joint space narrowing [68]. CT is more sensitive in detecting early joint space narrowing and subchondral sclerosis when compared with MR imaging, but MR imaging has been shown to demonstrate good agreement with CT with little clinically relevant difference [69,70]. In addition, MR imaging can demonstrate edema in the adjacent posterior elements and in the adjacent soft tissues (Fig. 12) [71].

Cysts near the facet joints may represent synovial cysts, ganglion cysts, or cysts of the ligamentum flavum. It is often difficult to distinguish these entities by radiologic, pathologic, or surgical means [72].

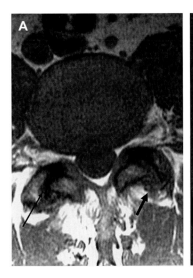 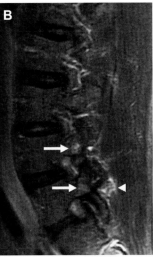

Fig. 12. Facet degeneration. (*A*) T1-weighted axial MR image demonstrates severe joint space narrowing associated with loss of normal cartilage signal (*thin black arrow*). Posterior osteophytes and capsular hypertrophy are also noted on this axial image (*thick black arrow*). (*B*) T2-weighted sagittal MR image with fat saturation demonstrates high signal in the adjacent pedicles (*thick white arrows*) and soft tissues adjacent to the facet joint (*white arrowhead*). This patient experienced profound improvement of his axial back pain after therapeutic facet injection.

Synovial cysts are not uncommon sequelae of facet arthropathy. In one review of 300 lumbar spine MR imaging studies, 7 patients (2.3%) had anterior facet cysts and 23 patients (7.3%) had posterior facet cysts [73]. Although facet cysts may occur at any level, they are found most commonly in the lower lumbar spine, and approximately 90% are found at the L4–5 level. Posterior facet cysts are usually asymptomatic because they project posteriorly into the paraspinal musculature. Anterior facet cysts may contribute to spinal canal or neural foraminal stenosis depending on the anterior location where these cysts are positioned (see Fig. 12). On CT imaging, facet cysts may be difficult to identify because their fluid density is similar to that of cerebrospinal fluid. Facet cysts may also have increased density secondary to hemorrhage or mural calcification and may have dramatically decreased signal because of intracystic gas. These factors are common in facet cysts and may aid in their detection. Facet cysts are amenable to percutaneous treatment [74] and will fill with contrast during facet joint injection (Fig. 13). In addition to the variable signal characteristics of the facet cysts seen on MR imaging, rim enhancement may be seen after administration of gadolinium. An extradural, well-marginated cystic mass near a site of facet arthropathy or spondylolisthesis strongly suggests the diagnosis of a facet joint cyst [74–76].

Degenerative changes of the interspinous ligament

Narrowing of the intervertebral disc may lead to abnormal contact between the dorsal spinous processes and degeneration of the interspinous ligaments and the adjacent spinous processes. These ligaments are normally low signal on T1- and T2-weighted images. As patients age, numerous changes can be seen in these ligaments, including fatty degeneration resulting in T1 shortening and increased cellularity resulting in T2 prolongation [77]. The clinical significance of these changes is unknown.

Interspinous pseudarthrosis formation and cyst formation can also occur secondary to close approximation of the spinous processes. This formation has been termed Baastrup's phenomenon (after a physician in the 1930s who initially recognized the clinical importance of the spinous process and adjacent soft tissues) and has been associated with clinically localized tenderness that is exacerbated with extension and relieved with flexion, anesthetic injections, or surgical excision [78]. Redundancy of the interspinous ligament may extend into the posterior aspect of the central spinal canal, resulting in effacement of the retrothecal fat pad and posterior narrowing of the spinal canal because of the redundant posterior ligamentous soft tissue. When the posterior degenerative changes are severe, a adventitial bursa may form and occasionally may communicate with the facet joints. Arthrography of the facets results in a butterfly appearance on a frontal view in this circumstance [79]. Interspinous bursae or hypertrophic degenerative changes can extend anteriorly from the interspinous space and can result in canal stenosis (Fig. 14) [80].

Complications of degenerative spinal disease

Scoliosis and kyphosis

Degenerative scoliosis most often occurs secondary to asymmetric degenerative change in a disc. The presence of the scoliosis leads to asymmetric

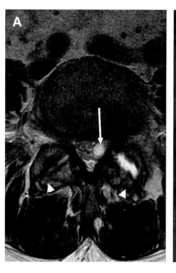 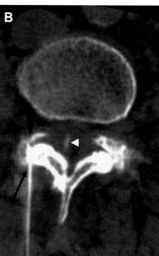

Fig. 13. Facet synovial cyst. (*A*) T2-weighted axial MR image demonstrates marked bilateral facet arthropathy (*white arrowheads*) with an associated left-sided synovial cyst (*white arrow*). (*B*) Axial CT image in another patient shows a needle placed in the right facet joint (*black arrow*) and contrast extending into a synovial cyst (*white arrowhead*) during therapeutic facet injection.

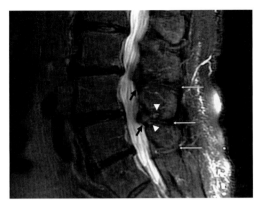

Fig. 14. Baastrup's phenomenon and associated spinal stenosis. T2-weighted sagittal MR image with fat saturation demonstrates close approximation of the dorsal spinous processes (*white arrows*) with subchondral cyst formation at the L4–5 junction (*white arrowheads*). Associated hypertrophic degenerative tissue (*black arrows*) extends anteriorly to contribute to canal stenosis.

loading of the spinal segment that already has degenerative changes present in the region of the increased asymmetric loading, which produces a positive feedback loop that tends to accelerate the degenerative changes in the region absorbing the most loading forces [81]. Progressive scoliosis can therefore appear in adult life without any precedence in adolescence, but degenerative changes superimposed on long-standing idiopathic curves may also present with a similar appearance. Several general characteristics of these types of curves help to distinguish between these two entities. Degenerative change leading to de novo scoliosis in adult life is usually short segment and most often occurs in the lumbar spine (Fig. 15). Loss of lordosis in the

lumbar spine is common and may be seen with acquired/degenerative scoliosis (see Fig. 15) [82]. Finally, spinal and foraminal stenoses are more commonly seen in scoliosis caused by degenerative changes, as compared with idiopathic scoliosis.

Thoracic kyphosis in adults is frequently secondary to disc degeneration. Asymmetric degenerative changes in the anterior portions of the disc may result in a kyphotic deformity (see Fig. 4). In a study of 1407 patients presenting with radiographic evidence of kyphosis, Schneider and colleagues [83] attributed 20% of kyphosis seen in the patients to osteoporotic compression fractures, compared with 50% attributed to degenerative changes.

Segmental instability

The initial event in degenerative vertebral instability is disc degeneration. This degeneration leads to narrowing of the disc space and buckling of the ligamentum flavum which can result in an unstable vertebral segment [84]. Resultant malalignment may manifest itself as anterior spondylolisthesis (anterolisthesis), posterior spondylolisthesis (retrolisthesis), rotational spondylolisthesis (rotolisthesis) or lateral spondylolisthesis, depending on the degree of degenerative change and on local anatomic factors. Degenerative retrolisthesis occurs classically secondary to disc degeneration and may result in spinal and foraminal stenosis. Anterolisthesis occurs most commonly at the L4–5 level and is usually secondary to facet osteoarthrosis. Degenerative rotational spondylolisthesis may occur secondary to asymmetric facet degeneration. Lateral spondylolisthesis and rotational spondylolisthesis are often seen in patients who have degenerative scoliosis.

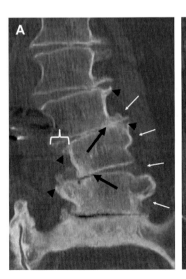
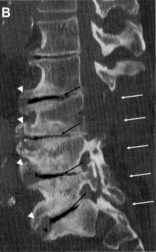

Fig. 15. Degenerative scoliosis: (*A*) Coronal CT reformatted image demonstrates levoscoliosis of the lower lumbar spine (*white arrows*). The image shows marked asymmetric disc degeneration (*black arrows*) and large lateral osteophytes (*black arrowheads*). Note the right lateral spondylolisthesis at L3–4 (*white bracket*). (*B*) Sagittal CT reformatted image shows loss of normal lumbar lordosis (*white arrows*) and severe degenerative disc disease at multiple levels (*black arrows*). Prominent anterior osteophytes are also present (*white arrowheads*).

Vertebral body movement may be seen on flexion and extension conventional radiographic views in the early stages of this process. Over time, secondary changes including hypertrophy of ligaments, facet osteoarthrosis, and osteophyte formation may develop. These secondary features can combine with the malalignment to result in narrowing of the spinal canal, lateral recesses, and neural foramina. Osteophytes have been shown to arise from increased spinal segment instability and the effectiveness of these osteophytes to stabilize spinal segment mobility in patients who have chronic spondylolisthesis has also been shown on kinematic MR imaging [85].

Spinal stenosis

Degenerative changes in the spine are the most common cause of spinal stenosis. Disc degeneration and loss of disc height typically result in a circumferential disc bulging, posterior bulging of a redundant posterior longitudinal ligament, and infolding/hypertrophy of the ligamentum flavum [86]. Late stages of intervertebral osteochondrosis are also associated with posterior osteophytes, which may cause further spinal canal narrowing. Patients who have symptomatic spinal stenosis, and especially those patients who present at a young age, often present with degenerative changes superimposed on some degree of congenital osseous canal narrowing.

The most concerning complication of cord compression is myelopathy. Myelopathy evolves over months to years, and results in demyelination, neuronal death, and increased MR imaging within the spinal cord (sometimes leading to cystic cavitation). The mechanism is poorly understood, but the initial insult is thought to be an increase in spinal cord pressure, caused by continuous or intermittent pinching of the cord, that results in chronic hypoperfusion. Surgery is often recommended in patients who have myelopathy to reduce the risks of permanent deficits and progressive symptoms [87]. Other investigators prefer conservative management and close follow-up, especially in mild cases [88]. Early diagnosis is important because many investigators consider surgery more effective early in the clinical course [89].

MR imaging is equivalent to CT myelography in the assessment of spinal stenosis, in the identification of the soft tissue or osseous compression of the spinal cord, and in the assessment of the thecal sac and neural foramina. MR imaging, however, offers the additional advantages of being less invasive and having no ionizing radiation, and it allows visualization of the neural structures including changes within the spinal cord itself. Increased intramedullary signal on the T2-weighted images is often seen in patients who have myelopathy and may indicate the presence of inflammatory edema, chronic ischemia, myelomalacia, or cystic cavitation [90]. Increased signal on the T2-weighted images is often subtle and enhancement on postgadolinium T1-weighted sequences may confirm the abnormality (Fig. 16).

MR imaging demonstrates only moderate agreement with clinical and electrophysiologic definitions of myelopathy. The absence of abnormal signal within the spinal cord signal changes does not rule out myelopathy. Significant clinical and electrophysiologic signs and symptoms may be present without an MR signal abnormality.

The anatomic presence of spinal stenosis in patients who are asymptomatic is not infrequent. Teresi and colleagues [91] found asymptomatic spinal stenosis in 16% of patients under 64 years old and

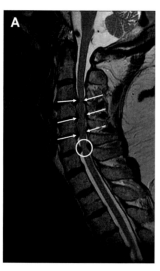
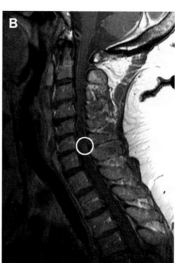

Fig. 16. Myelopathy. (*A*) Sagittal T2-weighted MR image with fat saturation demonstrates multiple levels of cord compression caused by anterior and posterior degenerative changes (*white arrows*). Intramedullary T2-prolongation is not convincingly seen on the T2-weighted images at the C6–7 level (*area within white circle*). (*B*) Sagittal postcontrast T1-weighted image shows abnormal enhancement in the spinal cord at the C6–7 level (*area within white circle*). This abnormal enhancement is consistent with myelopathy changes caused by the prominent spinal canal stenosis that is evident at that level.

in 26% of patients over 65 years old. Neither the degree of stenosis nor the presence of intramedullary signal changes is a reliable predictor on which to base the likelihood of the development of future symptoms in asymptomatic patients [91,92].

The significance of increased intramedullary signal on fluid-sensitive sequences is disputed. Some studies assert that increased intramedullary signal is a poor predictor of postoperative outcome in symptomatic patients [93,94], whereas others have not found it to predict either a negative or a positive outcome [88,95]. The added value of T1-weighted images may improve the prognostic value of MR imaging [96]. In general, low signal on the T1-weighted images suggests a poor prognosis, whereas increased T2 prolongation is nonspecific and can be seen in various clinical scenarios after surgical decompression. Surgery may still be advocated in patients with low T1 spinal cord signal change to prevent further deterioration.

Diffusion-weighted MR imaging may also be helpful in characterizing spinal cord abnormalities in patients who have myelopathy. Apparent diffusion coefficient (ADC) maps of the spine can show increased signal in affected areas of the spinal cord. In addition, diffusion tensor imaging can demonstrate increased magnitude in the transverse direction at the level of abnormality. These changes have been hypothesized to occur secondary to increased fluid within the interstitial spaces of the spinal cord, demyelination, and neuronal loss [97]. ADC maps and diffusion tensor imaging improved the sensitivity in detecting subtle changes, but at the cost of decreasing the specificity. The resultant high negative predictive value of this technique may be valuable in surgical decision making in patients in whom myelopathy is suspected. Facon and colleagues [98] examined 15 patients who had myelopathy and 11 controls with fractional anisotropy and ADC values. They found fractional anisotropy to be more sensitive and specific for myelopathy than either conventional T2-weighted MR imaging or ADC maps in this series. Larger studies are needed to confirm the results of this study but this early data may be of value when correctly applied in the appropriate clinical scenario.

Spinal cord and nerve root compression is a dynamic phenomenon that often worsens in an erect position or with certain movements. Conventional MR imaging occurs with the patient in a neutral, recumbent position. Conventional myelography, which may be performed in the upright or standing position, may demonstrate dynamic neural impingement that is only apparent on weight bearing or with provocative maneuvers. More recently, kinematic MR imaging has been advocated to assess for dynamic causes of neural compression [99,100]. Patients may be scanned in an open magnet while weight bearing. Previously occult abnormalities including disc herniations, infolding of ligamentous structures, subluxations, and traumatic injuries have all been demonstrated using this technique (Fig. 17).

Foraminal stenosis

Impingement of the nerve root may occur in the lateral recess or the neural foramen, or extraforaminally. Nerve root impingement is a common finding and is often asymptomatic. Correlation with symptoms of radiculopathy is essential. Lateral recess stenosis is best assessed on axial images. It is found most commonly at L4–5 and may be

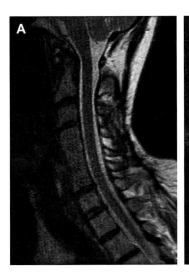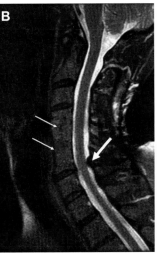

Fig. 17. Dynamic compression of the spine. (*A*) T2-weighted sagittal MR images in flexion in a patient who experienced symptoms of myelopathy with extension of the neck show no significant spinal canal narrowing. (*B*) T2-weighted sagittal MR images in extension show prominent bulging of posterior ligamentous structures resulting in significant stenosis at the C6–7 level (*thick white arrow*). Incidental note is made of previous C4–6 anterior vertebral body fusion (*thin white arrows*).

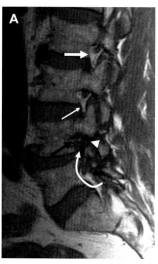
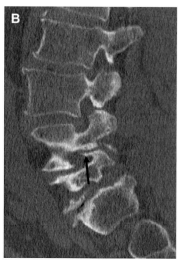

Fig. 18. Lumbar foraminal stenosis. (*A*) T1-weighted sagittal MR image demonstrates a normal neural foramen at the L2–3 level (*thick white arrow*). Mild foraminal narrowing is present at the L3–4 level (*thin white arrow*), primarily secondary to a posterior disc prominence and facet joint hypertrophic change. Severe stenosis is present at the L4–5 level (*thick black arrow*) because of facet arthropathy (*white arrowhead*), disc height loss, and disc bulging (*curved white arrow*). (*B*) Sagittal reformatted CT of the L4–5 foramen demonstrates collision osteophyte formation (*black arrow*) between the superior articular process of L5 and the pars interarticularis of L4. (The superior articular process and the pars inter-articularis structures are not well seen on this single sagittal image).

secondary to facet osteophytes, posterior ligamentous thickening, or a disc herniation.

Neural foraminal narrowing is most commonly caused by uncovertebral osteophytes in the cervical spine. Facet arthropathy is another common degenerative process that will produce neural foraminal narrowing. Loss of disc height contributes to foraminal stenosis by narrowing of the craniocaudal diameter. Restoration of disc height is an important component of most decompression surgeries. Lumbar neural foramina are typically well seen on both axial and sagittal MR imaging but the cervical neural foramina are best evaluated on the axial MR imaging sequences.

Degenerative facet changes and disc herniations are common causes of foraminal stenosis in the thoracic and lumbar spine. Neural foraminal narrowing in these regions may also result from decreased disc height, osteophytes from the disc space, and malalignment. Reduction of disc height can also result in contact of the superior articular process of the facet with the pars interarticularis and adjacent undersurface of the pedicle in the more superior vertebral segment (Fig. 18), which can result in collision osteophytes with additional narrowing of the superior aspect of the neural foramen. Pseudarthrosis and cyst formation may also occur secondary to this abnormal articulation, resulting in further neural foraminal and spinal canal narrowing [62].

Neural foraminal stenosis is best assessed on sagittal images in the thoracic and lumbar spine. The foramen has an ovoid formation and is filled with cerebrospinal fluid and fat. Mild foraminal narrowing is visualized on sagittal images as a "keyhole"-type appearance. Moderate narrowing effaces the inferior portion of the foramen at the level of the disc. Severe foraminal narrowing results in effacement of the fat in the foramen (see Fig. 18). Other signs of foraminal and spinal stenosis include loss of fat around the exiting nerves and thecal sac. Effacement of contrast or cerebrospinal fluid around nerve roots in the lumbar cistern is also an important sign. MR imaging with gadolinium may show inflammatory changes in and around an entrapped nerve root.

Summary

Degenerative changes of the spine may involve the disc space, the facet joints, or the supportive and surrounding soft tissues. MR imaging is an ideally suited modality for delineating the presence, extent, and complications of degenerative spinal disease. Other imaging modalities such as radiography, myelography, and CT may provide additional and complimentary information in selected cases. Percutaneous procedures such as discography and diagnostic injections may be used to confirm that a morphologic abnormality is the source of symptoms. Correlation with clinical and electrophysiologic data is also helpful for accurate diagnosis. Combining the information obtained from imaging studies with the patient's clinical presentation is mandatory for determining the appropriate patient management strategy, especially true in patients afflicted with any one of a number of conditions that are directly attributed to the degenerative processes of the spine.

References

[1] Cavanaugh JM, Ozaktay AC, Yamashita HT. King AI Lumbar facet pain: biomechanics, neuroanatomy and neurophysiology. J Biomech 1996;29(9):1117–29.

[2] Mooney V. Where is the pain coming from? Ann Med 1989;21(5):321–5.

[3] Schwarzer AC, Aprill CN, Derby R, et al. The relative contributions of the disc and zygapophyseal joint in chronic low back pain. Spine 1994;19(7):801–6.

[4] Matsumoto M, Fujimura Y, Suzuki N, et al. MRI of cervical intervertebral discs in asymptomatic subjects. J Bone Joint Surg Br 1998;80(1):19–24.

[5] Weishaupt D, Zanetti M, Hodler J, et al. MR imaging of the lumbar spine: prevalence of intervertebral disk extrusion and sequestration, nerve root compression, end plate abnormalities, and osteoarthritis of the facet joints in asymptomatic volunteers. Radiology 1998;209(3):661–6.

[6] Boden SD, McCowin PR, Davis DO, et al. Abnormal magnetic-resonance scans of the cervical spine in asymptomatic subjects. A prospective investigation. J Bone Joint Surg Am 1990;72(8):1178–84.

[7] Adams MA, Roughley PJ. What is intervertebral disc degeneration, and what causes it? Spine 2006;31(18):2151–61.

[8] Boos N, Weissbach S, Rohrbach H, et al. Classification of age-related changes in lumbar intervertebral discs: 2002 Volvo Award in Basic Science. Spine 2002;27(23):2631–44.

[9] Battie MC, Videman T, Parent E. Lumbar disc degeneration: epidemiology and genetic influences. Spine 2004;29(23):2679–90.

[10] Videman T, Battie MC. The influence of occupation on lumbar degeneration. Spine 1999;24(11):1164–8.

[11] Adams MA, Hutton WC. Prolapsed intervertebral disc. A hyperflexion injury 1981 Volvo Award in Basic Science. Spine 1982;7(3):184–91.

[12] Verzijl N, DeGroot J, Thorpe SR, et al. Effect of collagen turnover on the accumulation of advanced glycation end products. J Biol Chem 2000;275(50):39027–31.

[13] Pfirrmann CW, Metzdorf A, Zanetti M, et al. Magnetic resonance classification of lumbar intervertebral disc degeneration. Spine 2001;26(17):1873–8.

[14] Dillon WP, Kaseff LG, Knackstedt VE, et al. Computed tomography and differential diagnosis of the extruded lumbar disc. J Comput Assist Tomogr 1983;7(6):969–75.

[15] McAfee PC, Ullrich CG, Yuan HA, et al. Computed tomography in degenerative spinal stenosis. Clin Orthop Relat Res 1981;(161):221–34.

[16] Boutin RD, Steinbach LS, Finnesey K. MR imaging of degenerative diseases in the cervical spine. Magn Reson Imaging Clin N Am 2000;8(3):471–90.

[17] Osti OL, Vernon-Roberts B, Moore R, et al. Annular tears and disc degeneration in the lumbar spine. A post-mortem study of 135 discs. J Bone Joint Surg Br 1992;74(5):678–82.

[18] Hilton RC, Ball J. Vertebral rim lesions in the dorsolumbar spine. Ann Rheum Dis 1984;43(2):302–7.

[19] Stadnik TW, Lee RR, Coen HL, et al. Annular tears and disk herniation: prevalence and contrast enhancement on MR images in the absence of low back pain or sciatica. Radiology 1998;206(1):49–55.

[20] Ross JS, Modic MT, Masaryk TJ. Assessment of extradural degenerative disease with Gd-DTPA-enhanced MR imaging: correlation with surgical and pathologic findings. AJR Am J Roentgenol 1990;154(1):151–7.

[21] Aprill C, Bogduk N. High-intensity zone: a diagnostic sign of painful lumbar disc on magnetic resonance imaging. Br J Radiol 1992;65(773):361–9.

[22] Peng B, Hou S, Wu W, et al. The pathogenesis and clinical significance of a high-intensity zone (HIZ) of lumbar intervertebral disc on MR imaging in the patient with discogenic low back pain. Eur Spine J 2006;15(5):583–7.

[23] Munter FM, Wasserman BA, Wu HM, et al. Serial MR imaging of annular tears in lumbar intervertebral disks. AJNR Am J Neuroradiol 2002;23(7):1105–9.

[24] Schellhas KP, Pollei SR, Gundry CR, et al. Lumbar disc high-intensity zone. Correlation of magnetic resonance imaging and discography. Spine 1996;21(1):79–86.

[25] Kakitsubata Y, Theodorou DJ, Theodorou SJ, et al. Magnetic resonance discography in cadavers: tears of the annulus fibrosus. Clin Orthop Relat Res 2003;Feb(407):228–40.

[26] Saifuddin A, MSweeney E, Lehovsky J. Development of lumbar high intensity zone on axial loaded magnetic resonance imaging. Spine 2003;28(21):E449–51.

[27] Kluner C, Kivelitz D, Rogalla P, et al. Percutaneous discography: comparison of low-dose CT, fluoroscopy and MRI in the diagnosis of lumbar disc disruption. Eur Spine J 2006;15(5):620–6 [Epub 2005 Nov 16].

[28] Yoshida H, Fujiwara A, Tamai K, et al. Diagnosis of symptomatic disc by magnetic resonance imaging: T2-weighted and gadolinium-DTPA-enhanced T1-weighted magnetic resonance imaging. J Spinal Disord Tech 2002;15(3):193–8.

[29] Walsh TR, Weinstein JN, Spratt KF, et al. Lumbar discography in normal subjects. A controlled, prospective study. J Bone Joint Surg Am 1990;72(7):1081–8.

[30] Carragee EJ, Tanner CM, Yang B, et al. False-positive findings on lumbar discography. Reliability of subjective concordance assessment

during provocative disc injection. Spine 1999; 24(23):2542–7.

[31] Carragee EJ, Lincoln T, Parmar VS, et al. A gold standard evaluation of the "discogenic pain" diagnosis as determined by provocative discography. Spine 2006;31(18):2115–23.

[32] Fardon DF, Milette PC. Combined Task Forces of the North American Spine Society, American Society of Spine Radiology, and American Society of Neuroradiology. Nomenclature and classification of lumbar disc pathology. Recommendations of the Combined Task Forces of the North American Spine Society, American Society of Spine Radiology, and American Society of Neuroradiology. Spine 2001;26(5):E93–113.

[33] Modic MT, Ross JS, Masaryk TJ. Imaging of degenerative disease of the cervical spine. Clin Orthop Relat Res 1989;(239):109–20.

[34] Glickstein MF, Burke DL Jr, Kressel HY. Magnetic resonance demonstration of hyperintense herniated discs and extruded disc fragments. Skeletal Radiol 1989;18(7):527–30.

[35] Sengupta DK, Kirollos R, Findlay GF, et al. The value of MR imaging in differentiating between hard and soft cervical disc disease: a comparison with intraoperative findings. Eur Spine J 1999; 8(3):199–204.

[36] Ahn Y, Lee SH, Lee SC, et al. Factors predicting excellent outcome of percutaneous cervical discectomy: analysis of 111 consecutive cases. Neuroradiology 2004;46(5):378–84.

[37] Jarvik JG, Hollingworth W, Heagerty PJ, et al. Three-year incidence of low back pain in an initially asymptomatic cohort: clinical and imaging risk factors. Spine 2005;30(13):1541–8.

[38] Borenstein DG, O'Mara JW Jr, Boden SD, et al. The value of magnetic resonance imaging of the lumbar spine to predict low-back pain in asymptomatic subjects: a seven-year follow-up study. J Bone Joint Surg Am 2001;83(9): 1306–11.

[39] Chung CB, Vande Berg BC, Tavernier T, et al. End plate marrow changes in the asymptomatic lumbosacral spine: frequency, distribution and correlation with age and degenerative changes. Skeletal Radiol 2004;33(7):399–404.

[40] Fandino J, Botana C, Viladrich A, et al. Reoperation after lumbar disc surgery: results in 130 cases. Acta Neurochir (Wien) 1993;122(1–2): 102–4.

[41] Carragee EJ, Han MY, Suen PW, et al. Clinical outcomes after lumbar discectomy for sciatica: the effects of fragment type and annular competence. J Bone Joint Surg Am 2003;85(1): 102–8.

[42] Dora C, Schmid MR, Elfering A, et al. Lumbar disk herniation: do MR imaging findings predict recurrence after surgical diskectomy? Radiology 2005;235(2):562–7.

[43] Banerian KG, Wang AM, Samberg LC, et al. Association of vertebral end plate fracture with pediatric lumbar intervertebral disk herniation:

value of CT and MR imaging. Radiology 1990; 177(3):763–5.

[44] Wagner A, Albeck MJ, Madsen FF. Diagnostic imaging in fracture of lumbar vertebral ring apophyses. Acta Radiol 1992;33(1):72–5.

[45] Shirado O, Yamazaki Y, Takeda N, et al. Lumbar disc herniation associated with separation of the ring apophysis: is removal of the detached apophyses mandatory to achieve satisfactory results? Clin Orthop Relat Res 2005;(431):120–8.

[46] Asazuma T, Nobuta M, Sato M, et al. Lumbar disc herniation associated with separation of the posterior ring apophysis: analysis of five surgical cases and review of the literature. Acta Neurochir (Wien) 2003;145(6):461–6.

[47] Resnick D. Degenerative disease of the spine. Radiology 1985;156:3–14.

[48] Modic MT, Steinberg PM, Ross JS, et al. Degenerative disk disease: assessment of changes in vertebral body marrow with MR imaging. Radiology 1988;166(1 Pt 1):193–9.

[49] de Roos A, Kressel H, Spritzer C, et al. MR imaging of marrow changes adjacent to end plates in degenerative lumbar disk disease. AJR Am J Roentgenol 1987;149(3):531–4.

[50] Mitra D, Cassar-Pullicino VN, McCall IW. Longitudinal study of high intensity zones on MR of lumbar intervertebral discs. Clin Radiol 2004;59(11):1002–8.

[51] Toyone T, Takahashi K, Kitahara H, et al. Vertebral bone-marrow changes in degenerative lumbar disc disease. An MRI study of 74 patients with low back pain. J Bone Joint Surg Br 1994;76(5):757–64.

[52] Weishaupt D, Zanetti M, Hodler J, et al. Painful lumbar disk derangement: relevance of endplate abnormalities at MR imaging. Radiology 2001;218(2):420–7.

[53] Pfirrmann CW, Resnick D. Schmorl nodes of the thoracic and lumbar spine: radiographic-pathologic study of prevalence, characterization, and correlation with degenerative changes of 1,650 spinal levels in 100 cadavers. Radiology 2001;219(2):368–74.

[54] McFadden KD, Taylor JR. End-plate lesions of the lumbar spine. Spine 1989;14(8):867–9.

[55] Fahey V, Opeskin K, Silberstein M, et al. The pathogenesis of Schmorl's nodes in relation to acute trauma. An autopsy study. Spine 1998; 23(21):2272–5.

[56] Grive E, Rovira A, Capellades J, et al. Radiologic findings in two cases of acute Schmorl's nodes. AJNR Am J Neuroradiol 1999;20(9):1717–21.

[57] Wagner AL, Murtagh FR, Arrington JA, et al. Relationship of Schmorl's nodes to vertebral body endplate fractures and acute endplate disk extrusions. AJNR Am J Neuroradiol 2000;21(2): 276–81.

[58] Stabler A, Bellan M, Weiss M, et al. MR imaging of enhancing intraosseous disk herniation (Schmorl's nodes). AJR Am J Roentgenol 1997;168(4):933–8.

[59] Yilmazlar S, Kocaeli H, Uz A, et al. Clinical importance of ligamentous and osseous structures in the cervical uncovertebral foraminal region. Clin Anat 2003;16(5):404–10.

[60] Carrera GF, Haughton VM, Syvertsen A, et al. Computed tomography of the lumbar facet joints. Radiology 1980;134(1):145–8.

[61] Fujiwara A, Tamai K, Yamato M, et al. The relationship between facet joint osteoarthritis and disc degeneration of the lumbar spine: an MRI study. Eur Spine J 1999;8(5):396–401.

[62] Jinkins JR. Acquired degenerative changes of the intervertebral segments at and suprajacent to the lumbosacral junction. A radioanatomic analysis of the nondiskal structures of the spinal column and perispinal soft tissues. Radiol Clin North Am 2001;39(1):73–99.

[63] Dunlop RB, Adams MA, Hutton WC. Disc space narrowing and the lumbar facet joints. J Bone Joint Surg Br 1984;66(5):706–10.

[64] Fujiwara A, Tamai K, An HS, et al. Orientation and osteoarthritis of the lumbar facet joint. Clin Orthop Relat Res 2001;(385):88–94.

[65] el-Khoury GY, Renfrew DL. Percutaneous procedures for the diagnosis and treatment of lower back pain: diskography, facet-joint injection, and epidural injection. AJR Am J Roentgenol 1991;157(4):685–91.

[66] Fairbank JC, Park WM, McCall IW, et al. Apophyseal injection of local anesthetic as a diagnostic aid in primary low-back pain syndromes. Spine 1981;6(6):598–605.

[67] Schofferman J, Kine G. Effectiveness of repeated radiofrequency neurotomy for lumbar facet pain. Spine 2004;29(21):2471–3.

[68] Leonardi M, Biasizzo E, Fabris G, et al. CT evaluation of the lumbosacral spine. AJNR Am J Neuroradiol 1983;4(3):846–7.

[69] Leone A, Aulisa L, Tamburrelli F, et al. Ruolo della tomografia computerizzata e della risonanza magnetica nella valutazione della artropatia degenerativa delle facette articolari lombari. [The role of computed tomography and magnetic resonance in assessing degenerative arthropathy of the lumbar articular facets]. Radiol Med (Torino) 1994;88(5):547–52 [in Italian].

[70] Weishaupt D, Zanetti M, Boos N, et al. MR imaging and CT in osteoarthritis of the lumbar facet joints. Skeletal Radiol 1999;28(4):215–9.

[71] Morrison JL, Kaplan PA, Dussault RG, et al. Pedicle marrow signal intensity changes in the lumbar spine: a manifestation of facet degenerative joint disease. Skeletal Radiol 2000;29(12):703–7.

[72] Baker JK, Hanson GW. Cyst of the ligamentum flavum. Spine 1994;19(9):1092–4.

[73] Doyle AJ, Merrilees M. Synovial cysts of the lumbar facet joints in a symptomatic population: prevalence on magnetic resonance imaging. Spine 2004;29(8):874–8.

[74] Bureau NJ, Kaplan PA, Dussault RG. Lumbar facet joint synovial cyst: percutaneous treatment with steroid injections and distention–clinical and imaging follow-up in 12 patients. Radiology 2001;221(1):179–85.

[75] Liu SS, Williams KD, Drayer BP, et al. Synovial cysts of the lumbosacral spine: diagnosis by MR imaging. AJR Am J Roentgenol 1990;154(1):163–6.

[76] Jackson DE Jr, Atlas SW, Mani JR, et al. Intraspinal synovial cysts: MR imaging. Radiology 1989;170(2):527–30.

[77] Fujiwara A, Tamai K, An HS, et al. The interspinous ligament of the lumbar spine. Magnetic resonance images and their clinical significance. Spine 2000;25(3):358–63.

[78] Bywaters EG, Evans S. The lumbar interspinous bursae and Baastrup's syndrome. An autopsy study. Rheumatol Int 1982;2(2):87–96.

[79] Sarazin L, Chevrot A, Pessis E, et al. Lumbar facet joint arthrography with the posterior approach. Radiographics 1999;19(1):93–104.

[80] Chen CK, Yeh L, Resnick D, et al. Intraspinal posterior epidural cysts associated with Baastrup's disease: report of 10 patients. AJR Am J Roentgenol 2004;182(1):191–4.

[81] Aebi M. The adult scoliosis. Eur Spine J 2005; 14(10):925–48.

[82] Grubb SA, Lipscomb HJ, Coonrad RW. Degenerative adult onset scoliosis. Spine 1988; 13(3):241–5.

[83] Schneider DL, von Muhlen D, Barrett-Connor E, et al. Kyphosis does not equal vertebral fractures: the Rancho Bernardo study. J Rheumatol 2004;31(4):747–52.

[84] Herkowitz HN. Spine update. Degenerative lumbar spondylolisthesis. Spine 1995;20(9):1084–90.

[85] McGregor AH, Anderton L, Gedroyc WM, et al. The use of interventional open MRI to assess the kinematics of the lumbar spine in patients with spondylolisthesis. Spine 2002;27(14).

[86] Amundsen T, Weber H, Lilleas F, et al. Lumbar spinal stenosis. Clinical and radiologic features. Spine 1995;20(10):1178–86.

[87] Sampath P, Bendebba M, Davis JD, et al. Outcome of patients treated for cervical myelopathy. A prospective, multicenter study with independent clinical review. Spine 2000;25(6):670–6.

[88] Matsumoto M, Toyama Y, Ishikawa M, et al. Increased signal intensity of the spinal cord on magnetic resonance images in cervical compressive myelopathy. Does it predict the outcome of conservative treatment? Spine 2000;25(6):677–82.

[89] Matsuda Y, Shibata T, Oki S, et al. Outcomes of surgical treatment for cervical myelopathy in patients more than 75 years of age. Spine 1999;24(6):529–34.

[90] Mair WG, Druckman R. The pathology of spinal cord lesions and their relation to the clinical

features in protrusion of cervical intervertebral discs; a report of four cases. Brain 1953;76(1): 70–91.

[91] Teresi LM, Lufkin RB, Reicher MA, et al. Asymptomatic degenerative disk disease and spondylosis of the cervical spine: MR imaging. Radiology 1987;164(1):83–8.

[92] Bednarik J, Kadanka Z, Dusek L, et al. Presymptomatic spondylotic cervical cord compression. Spine 2004;29(20):2260–9.

[93] Takahashi M, Yamashita Y, Sakamoto Y, et al. Chronic cervical cord compression: clinical significance of increased signal intensity on MR images. Radiology 1989;173(1): 219–24.

[94] Wada E, Yonenobu K, Suzuki S, et al. Can intramedullary signal change on magnetic resonance imaging predict surgical outcome in cervical spondylotic myelopathy? Spine 1999; 24(5):455–61.

[95] Okais N, Moussa R, Hage P. Valeur de l'hypersignal a l'irm dans les myelopathies cervicarthrosiquesn. [Value of increased MRI signal intensity in cervical arthrosis in myelopathies].

Neurochirurgie 1997;43(5):285–90 [discussion: 290–1] [in French].

[96] Morio Y, Teshima R, Nagashima H, et al. Correlation between operative outcomes of cervical compression myelopathy and MRI of the spinal cord. Spine 2001;26(11):1238–45.

[97] Demir A, Ries M, Moonen CT, et al. Diffusion-weighted MR imaging with apparent diffusion coefficient and apparent diffusion tensor maps in cervical spondylotic myelopathy. Radiology 2003;229(1):37–43.

[98] Facon D, Ozanne A, Fillard P, et al. MR diffusion tensor imaging and fiber tracking in spinal cord compression. AJNR Am J Neuroradiol 2005;26(6):1587–94.

[99] Jinkins JR, Dworkin JS, Damadian RV. Upright, weight-bearing, dynamic-kinetic MRI of the spine: initial results. Eur Radiol 2005;15(9):1815–25.

[100] Muhle C, Resnick D, Ahn JM, et al. In vivo changes in the neuroforaminal size at flexion-extension and axial rotation of the cervical spine in healthy persons examined using kinematic magnetic resonance imaging. Spine 2001;26(13):E287–93.

MAGNETIC RESONANCE IMAGING CLINICS

ELSEVIER SAUNDERS

Magn Reson Imaging Clin N Am 15 (2007) 239–255

Primary Tumors of the Osseous Spine

Jorge A. Vidal, MD[a], Mark D. Murphey, MD[a,b],*

- Benign tumors of the osseous spine
  Enostosis
  Osteoid osteoma
  Osteoblastoma
  Giant cell tumor
  Aneurysmal bone cyst
  Osteochondroma
  Hemangioma
  Langerhans cell histiocytosis
- Malignant primary tumors of the osseous spine
  Chordoma
  Chondrosarcoma
  Ewing sarcoma and primitive neuroectodermal tumor
  Osteosarcoma
- Summary
- References

Primary tumors of the spine are infrequent lesions compared with metastatic disease, multiple myeloma, and lymphoma. MR imaging, commonly used to evaluate the spine in patients presenting with pain, can further characterize lesions that may be encountered on other imaging studies, such as radiographs, bone scintigraphy, or CT. It is of utmost importance that radiologists identify these lesions and guide referring physicians to the appropriate patient evaluation. Radiologists must also avoid providing an all-encompassing broad differential diagnosis list in situations where the clinical scenario or specific imaging features can significantly limit the diagnostic possibilities.

Benign tumors of the osseous spine

Enostosis

An enostosis, commonly referred to as a bone island, is a frequent benign tumor of the osseous

spine and is reported to be present in up to 14% of cadavers. These lesions are likely developmental and some consider them similar to hamartomas [1].

The most common locations are between T1 and T7 in the thoracic spine and between L2 and L3 in the lumbar spine. These lesions have a dense radiographic and CT appearance due to their histological composition of cortical bone. The margins of enostoses are usually irregular, appearing spiculated or thornlike, and commonly merge into the medullary or cancellous bone surrounding the lesion. These lesions are typically round to oval in shape and range in size between 2 mm to approximately 2 cm in diameter. Enostoses are often located adjacent to the endosteal surface of the cortex (Fig. 1).

Enostoses usually have normal radiotracer uptake on bone scintigraphy, although larger lesions may occasionally show mild increased radiotracer activity (33% of lesions show some degree of

a Department of Radiologic Pathology, Musculoskeletal Division, Armed Forces Institute of Pathology, 14th St. and Alaska Avenue, Washington, DC 20306-6000, USA
b Uniformed Services University of the Health Sciences, 4301 Jones Bridge Road, Bethesda, MD 20814, USA
* Corresponding author. Department of Radiologic Pathology, Musculoskeletal Division, Armed Forces Institute of Pathology, 14th St. and Alaska Ave., Washington, DC 20306-6000.
E-mail address: murphey@afip.osd.mil (M.D. Murphey).

increased radiotracer uptake) [2]. On MR imaging, enostoses demonstrate low signal on both T1-weighted images and T2-weighted images due to their lack of mobile protons (see Fig. 1). The differential considerations for a sclerotic spine lesion include osteoblastic metastases, osteoid osteoma, and low-grade osteosarcoma.

It is important to be able to recognize these lesions to avoid unnecessary evaluation. It may be difficult to distinguish enostoses from some osteoblastic metastases, particularly in large lesions. Enostoses, however, do not reveal significant increased tracer uptake. They have a thornlike margin, are typically solitary, and have normal adjacent trabecular bone, as opposed to osteoblastic metastases. These features allow differentiation of these lesions in the vast majority of cases and may obviate the need for biopsy. However, biopsy should be considered if there is an increase in size of more than 25% to 50% in a 6-month to 1-year period.

Conditions related to enostoses include osteopoikilosis, osteopathia striata, and melorheostosis.

Osteoid osteoma

Osteoid osteoma accounts for 11% of all biopsied primary bone tumors. Ten percent of the osteoid osteomas are located within the spine. These lesions are a common cause of painful scoliosis and may present with focal or radicular pain and, occasionally, with gait disturbances. These lesions may demonstrate symptoms that are worse at night and that are relieved by nonsteroidal anti-inflammatory drugs (NSAIDs). The pain may also be aggravated by the imbibition of alcohol. Young (10 to 20 years old) patients are most commonly affected and there is a male predilection (2:1–3:1) [3–5].

Osteoid osteomas are small (<1.5–2.0 cm in diameter) vascular lesions with well-organized, interconnected trabecular bone in a background of fibrous connective tissue. These lesions are frequently surrounded by a variable degree of reactive bone and are often associated with cortical thickening and bony sclerosis.

The lumbar spine is the most frequently affected portion of the spine (59% of lesions) followed by the cervical (27%), thoracic (12%), and sacral segments (2%). Spinal osteoid osteomas are located within the posterior elements of the vertebra (pedicles, superior and inferior articular processes, lamina, transverse, and spinous processes) in 93% of cases. The remaining lesions are located within the vertebral body [3,6].

Osteoid osteomas are often occult on radiographs owing to their small size (the lesion, by definition, is <1.5–2.0 cm in diameter), radiolucent appearance, and posterior element location. CT allows for optimal identification of the nidus and the central calcification is also frequently detected (Fig. 2). This central mineralization has a sequestrumlike appearance that could potentially be confused with other lesions that may have a sequestrum, including osteomyelitis, osteoblastic metastases, lymphoma, Langerhans cell histiocytosis (LCH), osteoblastoma, and malignant fibrous histiocytoma. Osteoid osteomas reveal a variable degree of surrounding sclerosis on conventional radiographs or CT. This sclerosis, when found in the pedicle, may cause a radiodense pedicle. The differential diagnosis for a dense pedicle includes osteoblastic metastases, enostosis, low-grade infection, chronic infection, lymphoma, or reactive sclerosis caused by a mechanical abnormality, such as spondylolysis or an absent contralateral pedicle. These lesions demonstrate marked increased radiotracer uptake on bone scintigraphy. A double-uptake scintigraphic pattern has been described with osteoid osteomas. This double-uptake pattern

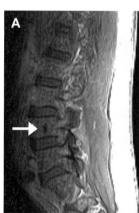
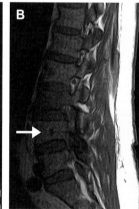
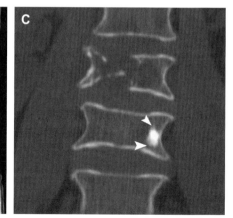

Fig. 1. Enostosis of L3. (*A*) Sagittal T1- and (*B*) T2-weighted MR images reveal low signal intensity (*white arrows*). (*C*) CT shows sclerotic lesion with thornlike margins (*white arrowheads*) abutting the cortex of the L3 vertebral body. These characteristics are typical of a bone island. Note the lytic lesion and pathologic fracture of L2.

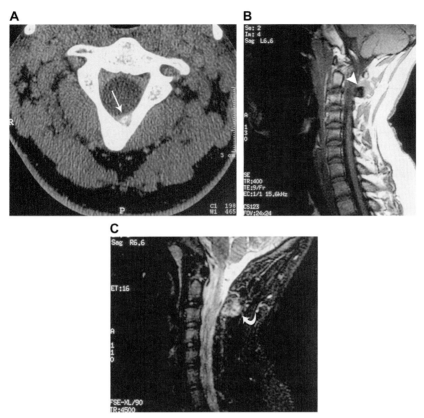

Fig. 2. Osteoid Osteoma of C2. (*A*) CT reveals nidus with central calcification in posterior left lamina of C2 (*white arrow*). (*B*) Sagittal T1-weighted MR image reveals subtle low signal intensity nidus (*white arrowhead*). (*C*) Prominent surrounding edema is seen on sagittal T2-weighted MR image (*curved arrow*).

is due to intense radionuclide uptake by the nidus, surrounded by less-intense activity of the osseous reaction structures.

MR imaging characteristics of the nidus include low to intermediate signal on T1-weighted images (see Fig. 2) and intermediate to high signal on T2-weighted images. This variable signal intensity is likely related to the degree of mineralization in the nidus. Surrounding reactive edema, both in the marrow and soft tissues, can be extensive, may obscure visualization of the nidus, and could initially suggest a more aggressive lesion (see Fig. 2). Chronically, the soft tissue edema can lead to muscle atrophy with increased adipose deposition.

Management for these lesions is quite variable. Although some favor medical management with NSAIDs, percutaneous image-guided ablation is commonly performed. Currently radio frequency ablation is the preferred method for appendicular lesions and has been used in the spine with some caution [7–10]. Laser and alcohol ablation are also accepted methods that may increase in use in the future [9,10]. Surgical excision is curative if the nidus is completely removed, but locating the lesion during operative intervention may be problematic.

Osteoblastoma

Osteoblastoma is a rare benign osteoid-producing tumor representing approximately 1% of all excised primary osseous tumors. This lesion has also been referred to as giant osteoid osteoma and osteogenic fibroma. Osteoblastomas commonly affect the vertebral column (30%–40% of cases) and are most frequently centered in the posterior elements (85% of lesions) with 42% extending into the vertebral body. Osteoblastomas are uncommonly confined to the vertebral body. Osteoblastomas usually present in young adults between the second and third decades of life, although cases have been reported as early as 3 years old and as late as 72 years of age. There is a mild male predominance (2:1) [11]. Clinically these lesions may present with dull localized pain. Neurological symptoms, however, are not uncommon and may include paresthesias, paraparesis, or paraplegia.

Osteoblastomas' imaging appearance can be divided into three categories or patterns: a tumor with a central radiolucent area and surrounding osseous sclerosis (similar to an osteoid osteoma, but greater than 1.5 to 2 cm in diameter); an expansile lesion with multiple small calcifications and a peripheral sclerotic rim (most common appearance in the spine); and a tumor with osseous expansion, bone destruction, infiltration of the surrounding soft tissues, and intermixed matrix calcification (this is a more aggressive pattern and the mineralization may have a chondroid appearance) [11–16]. These lesions demonstrate marked radiotracer uptake on bone scintigraphy similar to that associated with osteoid osteomas. CT shows areas of mineralization, expansile bone remodeling, and, frequently, sclerosis or a thin osseous shell about the lesion margins (Fig. 3).

MR imaging reveals a more varied appearance with no characteristic features. Nonspecific marrow replacement with low to intermediate signal intensity is seen on T1 weighting (see Fig. 3). The signal intensity on T2 weighting is variable, although in the authors' experience, low to intermediate signal intensity often predominates, likely related to the presence of osteoid (mineralized or unmineralized). Expansile remodeling of bone and soft tissue components may also be apparent and are optimally depicted by MR imaging. Surrounding marrow and soft tissue edema is generally less extensive compared with that seen in osteoid osteoma, although this feature is typically present and may lead to overestimation of lesion size [17]. Aneurysmal bone cyst (ABC) components are present in 10% to 15% of cases and demonstrate low signal on the T1-weighted images, marked high signal on the T2-weighted images, and multiple fluid levels.

Histologically, these lesions have similar features to osteoid osteoma and demonstrate interconnecting trabecular bone with an underlying fibrovascular stroma. Often osteoblastoma and osteoid osteoma are identical histologically and the specific entity distinction is based on size criteria with lesions greater than 2.0 cm designated as osteoblastomas.

Surgical resection is the treatment of choice with a recurrence rate of 10% to 15% for conventional osteoblastomas [11,13,16]. A subtype of these lesions histologically is aggressive osteoblastoma, which may correspond to more aggressive features radiologically as well. Aggressive osteoblastoma is an important designation because these lesions have a much higher rate of local recurrence (approaching 50%) than that of conventional

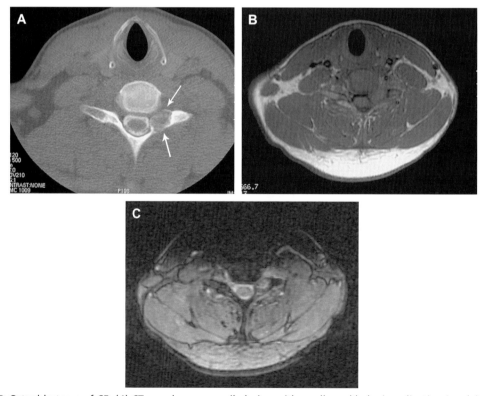

Fig. 3. Osteoblastoma of C5. (*A*) CT reveals an expansile lesion with small speckled mineralization involving the lamina of C5 (*arrows*). MR imaging demonstrates low to intermediate signal on both (*B*) axial T1- and (*C*) gradient echo images. Matrix mineralization cannot be identified on MR imaging.

osteoblastomas [13]. Multiple local recurrences of aggressive osteoblastoma can eventually lead to patient demise because of involvement of vital adjacent structures. Rarely, aggressive osteoblastoma may undergo malignant transformation to osteosarcoma and metastasize.

Giant cell tumor

Giant cell tumor (GCT), although commonly thought of as an appendicular lesion, can present in the spine (7% to 15% of all cases) representing the fourth most frequent location. The sacrum is the most commonly affected spinal area, followed by the thoracic, cervical, and lumbar segments in descending frequency [18–20]. There is a mild female predominance (3:2) and GCT usually presents in the second to fourth decade of life [21–23]. Clinical manifestations may include pain (often with a radicular distribution), weakness, and sensory deficits. These lesions may show a dramatic increase in size during pregnancy, presumably due to hormonal stimulation.

GCT is characterized as an expansile lesion with bone lysis. There is no evidence of mineralized matrix within these lesions. GCT of the sacrum is frequently centered in the S1-2 segment, presents with destruction of the sacral foramina, and commonly involves both sides of midline. Lesion extension across the sacroiliac joint is not rare [24]. In the mobile portion of the spine superior to the sacrum and inferior to the sphenooccipital region, GCT usually affects the vertebral body with extension into the posterior elements and paraspinal soft tissues. Associated vertebral collapse may also occur. GCT may also rarely involve the adjacent intervertebral disks and may extend into the adjacent vertebra. These lesions are usually vascular (75%–90% of cases). Bone scintigraphy may demonstrate a donut sign with increased radiotracer uptake around the periphery (57%) or diffusely increased radiotracer uptake. MR imaging reveals low to intermediate signal intensity on the T1-weighted and T2-weighted images (90%–95% of lesions), which is atypical for most osseous neoplasms (Fig. 4). GCT may demonstrate fluid–fluid levels on CT or MR imaging due to ABC components (see Fig. 4). These areas should be avoided during biopsy as they do not harbor diagnostic tissue.

Histologically, GCTs demonstrate abundant osteoclastic giant cells intermixed throughout a mononuclear spindle cell stroma. Similar to the imaging appearance, these lesions may contain ABC areas microscopically. Regions of previous hemorrhage with hemosiderin and prominent areas of fibrous tissue (high in collagen content, where giant cells are uncommon) may also be seen.

GCT is usually treated with curettage and cryosurgery or en bloc resection and bone graft. Local recurrence rates range between 2% and 25% but cryosurgery has been associated with improved disease-free periods [25]. The recurrence rate does not correspond to radiologic or microscopic appearance. Osseous recurrence usually presents as new bone destruction. GCT may also recur in the soft tissues and can rarely calcify or ossify about its periphery. GCT is one of the few benign tumors that may metastasize to the lungs (2%–5%) with about half of these metastatic lesions having a benign histology. Malignant GCT accounts for 5% to 7% of lesions, although in the authors' experience this percentage represents a significant overestimate of its true incidence. Many spinal lesions may be only partially resected because of their anatomic association with neurologic structures critical to normal

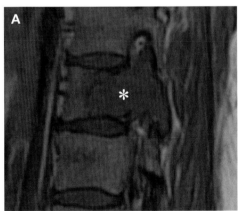 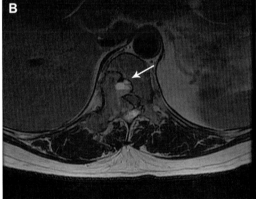

Fig. 4. Giant cell tumor of T11. (*A*) Sagittal T1-weighted MR image reveals marrow replacement (*asterisk*) centered in the vertebral body with posterior element extension. (*B*) In axial T2-weighted MR image, a small secondary aneurysmal bone cyst component reveals high signal intensity and fluid levels on the long TR image (*arrow*). The signal intensity on both images is predominantly intermediate.

functioning. In these cases, radiation therapy is often employed as an adjuvant. One of the risks of using radiation therapy in these cases is the later development of radiation-induced sarcoma.

Aneurysmal bone cyst

ABC typically affects young patients (younger than 20 years of age) with a mild female predilection [26]. The spine is involved in approximately 12% to 30% of cases, with the thoracic spine being the most frequently affected segment. Lumbar and cervical segments are affected less commonly. Sacral involvement, while rare, is usually centered in upper segments, similar to sacral involvement with GCT. Clinical presentation usually involves back pain or neurologic symptoms due to encroachment on the spinal canal or nerve roots.

Radiographically, spinal ABCs generally show marked expansile remodeling of bone and are typically centered in the posterior elements, although extension into the vertebral body is frequent (75%–90% of cases) [26]. Bone scintigraphy often demonstrates peripheral increased uptake of radionuclide (the donut sign) [1]. MR imaging and CT characteristics of primary ABC show single or, more commonly, multiple fluid levels comprising the entire lesion. The fluid–fluid levels within ABCs are indicative of hemorrhage with sedimentation [27]. As in other spinal lesions, MR imaging is valuable in determining the extent of the lesion and the relationship to the central canal and nerve roots. Supine positioning for approximately 10 minutes may be necessary to detect fluid levels by CT or MR imaging. The T1- or T2-weighted MR images may show increased signal due to methemoglobin within the fluid components (Fig. 5). The identification of fluid levels should initiate a search for a solid component indicative of a lesion (usually GCT or osteoblastoma) with a secondary ABC. ABC typically demonstrates a low signal intensity rim on all pulse sequences, which corresponds to an intact and often thickened periosteal

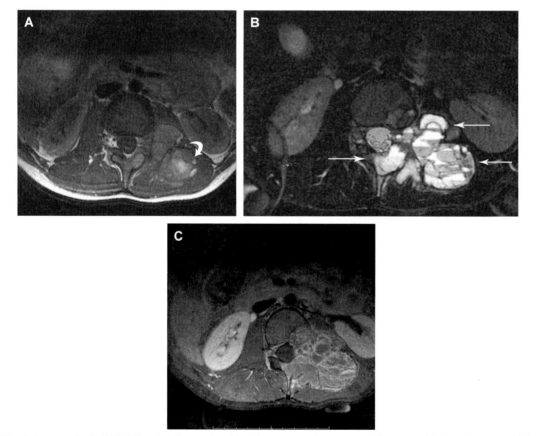

Fig. 5. Primary ABC of L2. (*A*) Axial T1-weighted MR image reveals an expansile mass with focal areas of high signal intensity representing hemorrhage (*curved arrow*). (*B*) Axial T2-weighted MR image demonstrates extensive fluid levels (*arrows*) throughout all components of the lesion. (*C*) An axial postcontrast MR image shows only mild peripheral and septal pattern of enhancement without solid components. The lesion is centered in the posterior elements with vertebral body extension.

membrane. Contrast enhancement of ABC is usually seen as a thin rim-and-septal pattern (see Fig. 5), whereas solid components in a secondary ABC enhance diffusely.

The imaging findings closely resemble the histologic appearance of this tumor. Primary ABCs have a characteristic appearance consisting of multiloculated blood-filled spaces. These blood-filled spaces are not lined by endothelium and thus do not represent vascular channels and are separated by thin septa. The septa interposed between the blood-filled spaces are composed of fibrous tissue, giant cells, and reactive bone.

Treatment of spinal ABCs may lead to high morbidity because vitally important neurologic structures (including nerve roots and the spinal cord) can be injured in the process. The overall recurrence rate for these lesions is 20% to 30% and may increase with incomplete resection [26,28]. The mainstay surgical therapy for ABCs is curettage and bone grafting [28]. Endovascular embolization, sclerotherapy, and percutaneous placement of polymethylmethacrylate have been reported with some success in the treatment of ABCs. These therapies can be occasionally employed to avoid radical surgery with rigid fixation [29,30].

Osteochondroma

Osteochondroma is an uncommon tumor in the spine comprising only 1% to 4% of solitary exostoses and 4% of all solitary spinal tumors. Even in cases of hereditary multiple exostoses (HME), only 7% to 9% of patients demonstrate an osteochondroma in the spine. These lesions are usually discovered during the third and fourth decades of life when solitary and a decade earlier in patients with HME. Solitary lesions may present with myelopathy in 34% of patients, while as many as 77% of patients present with these symptoms when multiple lesions are present [31–35]. Osteochondromas may be found anywhere along the spine. However, they appear to have a predilection for the cervical spine (particularly C2) [1]. Because of the associated neurological symptoms, lesions protruding into the spinal canal (Fig. 6) or impinging on the nerve roots are often discovered earlier when they are smaller, while lesions projecting posteriorly are usually larger and detected later due to the presence of a palpable mass [31–35].

Unlike appendicular lesions, osteochondromas of the spine are often occult on radiographs because of the complex osseous anatomy and frequent small size of lesions. MR imaging characteristics reveal a tumor with cancellous and cortical continuity with the bone from which it originates. The continuity of the marrow and cortical portions of the bone from which it originates is pathognomonic, but it can be difficult to demonstrate in small lesions. Lesions that are difficult to visualize either due to their location or their small size are frequently best evaluated with thin-section multiplanar CT (Fig. 7). A small hyaline cartilage cap (low to intermediate signal on T1-weighted images and high signal intensity on T2-weighted images) is usually apparent (see Fig. 7). A cartilage cap more than 1.5 cm thick in adults is worrisome for malignant transformation to a chondrosarcoma.

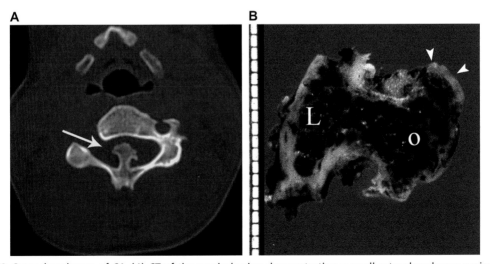

A   **B**

Fig. 6. Osteochondroma of C4. (*A*) CT of the cervical spine demonstrating a small osteochondroma projecting into the central canal at the level of C4 (*arrow*). (*B*) Photograph of sectioned gross specimen reveals marrow and cortical continuity between lamina (*L*) and the osteochondroma (*o*) as well as the small cartilage cap (*arrowheads*).

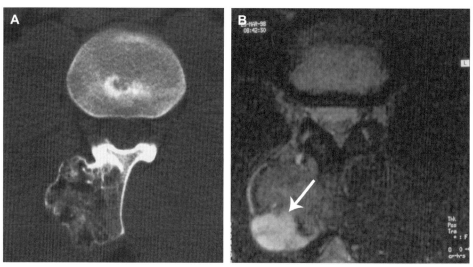

Fig. 7. Osteochondroma of L3. (*A*) CT reveals marrow and cortical continuity with the posterior elements of the lumbar spine, pathognomonic of an osteochondroma. (*B*) Axial T2-weighted MR imaging demonstrates increased signal in the hyaline cartilage cap (*arrow*).

Surgical excision with resection at the point of cortical and marrow continuity to the underlying bone is usually curative with improvement of symptoms seen in 89% of patients [31,36]. Incomplete resection can occasionally lead to recurrence, although this is unusual [1,31,36].

Hemangioma

Hemangioma of the spine is frequent, seen in as many as 11% of spines at autopsy. Multifocal lesions are present in 25% to 30% of cases [37]. Lesions occur most frequently in the thoracic spine, but may be present at any spinal level [38]. Radiographically, hemangiomas reveal prominent vertical trabeculae, which have been classically described as "corduroy" in appearance. These vertical, prominent trabeculae give the appearance of multiple punctate areas of sclerosis on axial CT images, creating the "polka dot" vertebra. Areas of decreased attenuation representing fatty stroma and serpentine vascular channels are also common. The MR imaging appearance of these lesions may also demonstrate fat overgrowth, seen as isointense to subcutaneous adipose tissue on T1- and T2-weighted images (Fig. 8). The polka-dot or corduroy appearance may also be seen on axial and sagittal/coronal MR images, respectively, as low signal intensity regions. However, this appearance is usually best

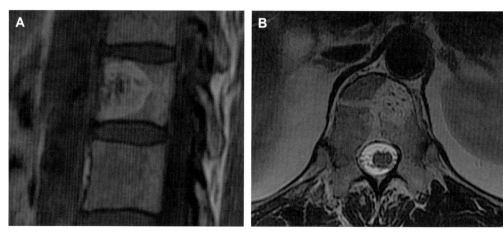

Fig. 8. Hemangioma of L2. (*A*) Sagittal T1-weighted and (*B*) axial T2-weighted MR images demonstrate signal intensity similar to retroperitoneal fat. Low signal intensity areas represent vascular channels and thickened trabeculae within this lesion.

appreciated on radiography or CT. The vascular components of these lesions demonstrate high signal intensity on T2-weighted images, reflecting slow blood flow and may reveal a serpentine pattern.

Histologically, hemangiomas represent a collection of thin-walled endothelial-lined blood vessels interspersed between nonvascular components, such as fat, muscle, fibrous tissue, or bone. These features correlate with the imaging findings. Multiple types (capillary, cavernous, arteriovenous, and venous) have been described, with the capillary type being the most common [39].

The vast majority of vertebral hemangiomas are incidentally discovered on routine MR imaging examinations. Hemangiomas with extension into the posterior elements, with paraspinal involvement and without a large amount of intertrabecular fatty stroma, are more likely to be associated with symptoms [40]. Neurological complaints and radiculopathy are frequently seen in patients who are symptomatic [40–43]. Large hemangiomas that weaken the vertebral bodies can result in fractures (Fig. 9), an obvious source of pain. Current treatment for symptomatic vertebral hemangiomas include endovascular embolization, vertebrectomy, sclerotherapy, and vertebroplasty [41].

Langerhans cell histiocytosis

LCH is a benign lesion that can affect the spine in 6% of cases [44]. The classic presentation of vertebra plana is seen in only approximately 15% of spinal LCH [45]. Partial vertebral collapse and focal marrow replacement are more commonly seen. A characteristic appearance of vertebral involvement

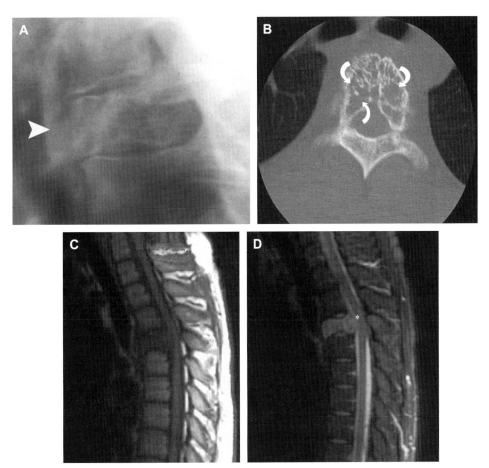

Fig. 9. Symptomatic hemangioma of T6. (*A*) Lateral thoracic spine radiograph demonstrates a compression deformity at the level of T6 (*arrowhead*) with abnormal trabecular pattern. (*B*) CT reveals the polka-dot appearance of hemangiomas and serpentine vascular channels (*curved arrows*). (*C*) Sagittal T1-weighted MR image and (*D*) T2-weighted MR image reveal marrow replacement and high signal intensity on the long TR sequence with a compression deformity of T6 and mild retropulsion into the spinal canal (*asterisk* in *D*). Vascular channels and trabecular thickening are much more apparent on CT than on MR imaging.

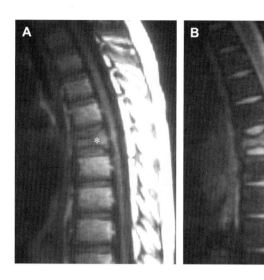

Fig. 10. Langerhans cell histiocytosis of T7. Sagittal T1-weighted MR image (A) shows marrow replacement (*) and increased signal intensity on sagittal T2-weighting (B). Note that there is collapse of the vertebral body with preservation of the endplates on all pulse sequences. No soft tissue mass is present.

with LCH is that the endplates are not involved. In the spine, the thoracic segments are most commonly affected, followed by the lumbar and cervical regions [46].

Radiologically, LCH demonstrates focal lytic lesions, which may progress to uniform vertebral collapse [44]. Bone scintigraphy shows increased uptake of radionuclide related to osteoblastic

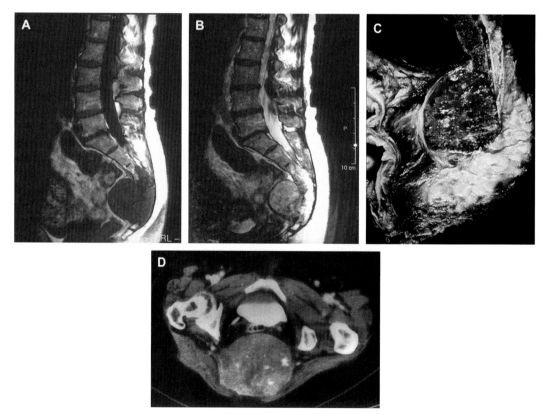

Fig. 11. Sacral chordoma with gross pathologic correlation. Sagittal T1-weighted MR image (A) demonstrates low signal intensity representing marrow replacement in a lesion centered at the level of S4 involving S3 and S5 and intermediate signal on T2-weighting (B). Photograph of a sagittal section from a gross specimen (C) demonstrates identical features corresponding to areas of marrow replacement. CT (D) reveals punctate mineralization within lesion.

activity. However, purely osteolytic lesions can be photopenic on nuclear scintigraphy [46]. The MR imaging appearance of LCH reveals areas of low signal marrow replacement on T1-weighted images (Fig. 10) and increased signal intensity on T2-weighted images (see Fig. 10). Small areas of soft tissue extension may be seen and surrounding hematoma may occur subsequent to vertebral collapse. MR imaging is useful in determining whether the disease is active or inactive (seen as vertebral body deformity without abnormal signal intensity). Therapeutic options include low-dose radiotherapy, steroid injections, chemotherapy, and surgical curettage [44–48]. LCH can be self-limiting if involvement is restricted to bone and may not require active treatment [44], but close observation is necessary to exclude progression of disease.

Malignant primary tumors of the osseous spine

Chordoma

Chordoma is the most common nonlymphoproliferative primary malignant neoplasm of the spine in adults. It has a peak incidence in the fifth decade of life and commonly presents in middle-aged patients (30–60 years old). This tumor is derived from notochordal remnants that extend from Rathke's pouch to the coccyx. Chordomas are almost exclusively seen in the midline with approximately 50% localized to the sacrum and 35% localized to the clivus. Unlike GCT, sacral chordomas are most frequently centered in the lower sacrum (S3-S4). The remaining 15% of lesions affect the mobile spinal segments, particularly the cervical region [49–53]. Rarely, chordomas arise in a paracentral location, which is along the spine in the soft tissues. These tumors have been described as "parachordoma."

Bone destruction predominates in spinal chordomas, although sclerosis in lesions involving the mobile portions of the spine can be seen in 15% of cases. Radiographs and CT frequently (64% of cases) [54] reveal intratumoral calcification in sacrococcygeal lesions (Fig. 11). Chordomas originating in the spine almost invariably extend into the paraspinal soft tissues laterally, dorsally, or ventrally and are associated with large associated masses. The

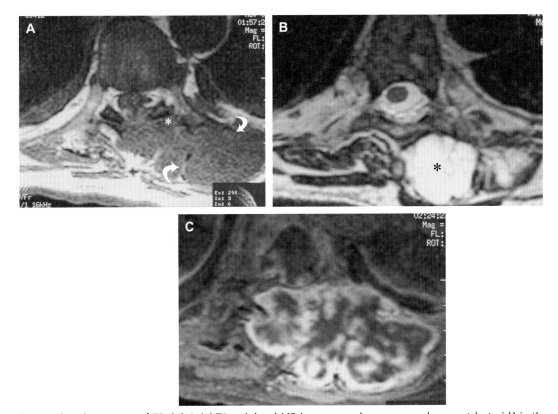

Fig. 12. Chondrosarcoma of T8. (*A*) Axial T1-weighted MR image reveals marrow replacement (*asterisk*) in the posterior elements with a large soft tissue component (*curved arrows*) and intermediate signal intensity. (*B*) Axial T2-weighted MR image demonstrates areas of marked increased signal intensity in the soft tissue component (*asterisk*) corresponding to cartilage with high water content. (*C*) Axial postcontrast MR image shows peripheral and septal enhancement of both osseous and soft tissue components typical of cartilaginous neoplasms.

series by Sung and colleagues [55] revealed sacroiliac joint involvement in 23% of cases. Chordomas show low to intermediate signal intensity on T1-weighted images and very high signal intensity on T2-weighted images due to a high water content (similar to that associated with the nucleus pulposus) (see Fig. 11). However, the lesions in the spheno-occipital region and intracranial chordomas may display increased signal on T1-weighted images due to a high protein content (rare in spinal chordomas) [54,56–58]. Lobular margins and foci of hemorrhage are also common in the authors' experience. Enhancement after administration of contrast is usually in a thick peripheral and septal pattern. This pattern is similar to, but more prominent than, the peripheral–septal enhancement seen with chondrosarcoma.

The location of the lesion usually determines the patient's prognosis (dependent on the ability to completely resect the tumor). Sacrococcygeal lesions have an improved survival rate (owing to their increased resectability), usually double that of chordomas at other sites [57].

Chondrosarcoma

Chondrosarcoma is the second most common non-lymphoproliferative primary malignant tumor of the spine in adults, accounting for 7% to 12% of these lesions. The spine represents the primary site in 3% to 12% of chondrosarcomas [59]. Presenting clinical symptoms are usually pain, palpable mass, and neurologic symptoms (45% of patients). Men are affected two to four times more frequently than women, and the mean age of patients

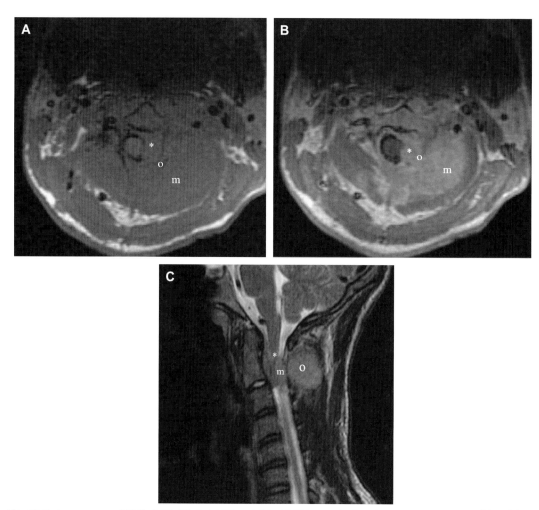

Fig. 13. Ewing-sarcoma–PNET of C4. (*A*) Axial T1-weighted MR image before intravenous contrast. (*B*) Axial T1-weighted MR image after intravenous contrast. (*C*) Sagittal T2-weighted MR image. Images demonstrate intermediate signal intensity on all pulse sequences and diffuse, moderate enhancement. (*m*) Soft tissue components have invaded the spinal canal (*asterisk*). (*o*) Large osseous components.

presenting with a chondrosarcoma is 45 years. Although these tumors can be seen at any level of the spine, the thoracic segments are the most commonly affected.

Histologically, most spinal chondrosarcomas are low-grade lesions. Common features include lobules of hyaline cartilage separated by fibrovascular septa, presence of myxoid tissue, and encasement of bone.

Radiologically, there is destruction of the osseous structures and frequent involvement of the posterior elements (40%), although lesions may be centered either anteriorly or posteriorly within the spine [60,61]. Mineralized matrix (typically with a ring-and-arc pattern) is best appreciated on radiographs or CT [59]. Chondrosarcoma typically demonstrates low signal intensity on T1-weighted images (Fig. 12) and high signal intensity on T2-weighted images. The lobular areas of hyaline cartilage growth are best demonstrated on T2-weighted images (see Fig. 12), while postcontrast images

frequently reveal a peripheral and septal enhancement pattern (characteristic of lobular, cartilage-rich lesions) on both MR imaging (see Fig. 12) and CT. Areas of matrix mineralization reveal low signal intensity on all pulse sequences and thus long TR pulse images frequently demonstrate prominent heterogeneity.

Treatment for spinal chondrosarcoma is surgical resection when possible. Because of lesion location and size, however, complete resection may not be possible without significant morbidity. Incomplete resection frequently leads to recurrence and eventual patient demise in 74% of cases [59]. Neither chemotherapy nor radiation is typically employed in treatment of chondrosarcoma.

Ewing sarcoma and primitive neuroectodermal tumor

Ewing sarcoma and primitive neuroectodermal tumor (PNET) are now considered similar and indistinct entities with very similar characteristics

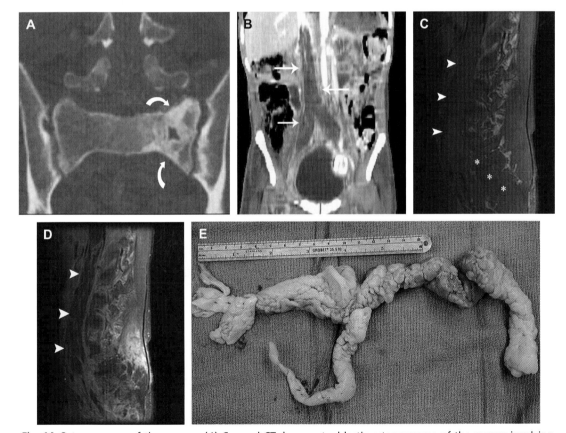

Fig. 14. Osteosarcoma of the sacrum. (*A*) Coronal CT shows osteoblastic osteosarcoma of the sacrum involving the left ala (*curved arrows*). (*B*) Coronal postcontrast CT reveals a large thrombus extending from the iliac veins to the right atrium (*arrows*). Sagittal T1-weighted MR images (*C*) before and (*D*) after contrast demonstrate marrow replacement (*asterisks* in *C*) of the sacral lesion and a large inferior vena cava tumor thrombus with intermixed areas of enhancement (*arrowheads*). (*E*) Photograph of gross specimen corresponding to the resected tumor thrombus.

Table 1: **Some imaging features of primary tumors of the spine**

Tumor	Age of presentation	Location on spine	Intensity of T1-weighted signal	Intensity of T2-weighted signal	Contrast enhancement	Characteristic features
				MR imaging		
Enostosis	Any age	Adjacent to endosteal surface of cortex	Low	Low	None	Thorny margins; normal adjacent trabecular bone
Osteoid osteoma	10–20y	Posterior elements 75%	Low	Intermediate	Diffuse, marked	Nidus; surrounding edema
Osteoblastoma	10–30y	Posterior elements 85%	Low to intermediate	Low to intermediate	Diffuse, variable degree	Expansile remodeling; multifocal mineralization; secondary ABC
Giant cell tumor	20–40y	Sacrum, vertebral body	Intermediate	Low to intermediate	Diffuse, moderate	Expansile remodeling; secondary ABC;
Aneurysmal bone cyst	<20y	Thoracic spine, posterior elements	Intermediate	Intermediate to high	Mild peripheral, septal	fluid levels expansile; no soft tissue component
Osteochondroma	20–40y	Cervical spine, C2	Same as vertebra	Same as vertebra	Same as vertebra	Marrow continuity; cartilage cap
Hemangioma	Any age	Vertebral body	High	High	Diffuse, moderate	Prominent trabeculae; serpentine channels; often follows fat signal
Langerhans cell histiocytosis	<20y	Vertebral body	Low to intermediate	High	Diffuse, moderate	Intact endplates; vertebra plana
Chordoma	30–60y	Sacrum 50%; clivus 35%	Low to intermediate	Very high	Peripheral, septal	Midline; destructive; calcification; soft tissue mass
Chondrosarcoma	40–50y	Thoracic spine	Low	High	Marked, peripheral, septal	Destructive; chondroid mineralization; soft tissue mass
Ewing-sarcoma–PNET	10–30y	Sacrococcygeal region	Intermediate	Intermediate to high	Diffuse, moderate	Destructive; soft tissue mass
Osteosarcoma	30–40y	Lumbosacral segments	Low	Low	Diffuse, moderate	Destructive; osteoid mineralization; soft tissue mass

pathologically, clinically, and radiologically. This family of neoplasms are the most common non-lymphoproliferative primary malignant tumors of the spine in children and adolescents with a mild male predilection [59,62–66]. Lesions of the spine account for 3% to 10% of all primary sites of Ewing-sarcoma–PNET [59,66]. Metastatic foci of Ewing-sarcoma–PNET involving the spine, however, are much more common than primary lesions. The most common location for primary Ewing-sarcoma–PNET lesions is the sacrococcygeal region, followed by the lumbar spine and the thoracic spine with only rare involvement of the cervical spine [62,64,66,67].

Histologically, Ewing-sarcoma–PNET is composed of small, round, blue cells with large irregular sheets of cells divided by septa, scant cytoplasm, and abundant collagen. Areas of necrosis are frequent in spinal lesions [68].

Radiologically, these tumors have a varied appearance, with the vast majority of lesions demonstrating aggressive bone lysis [59,66,69–71]. Vertebra plana has also been reported and extension to adjacent vertebral bodies can occur. Soft tissue involvement with large paraspinal masses is common and enlargement of these masses can lead to spinal canal invasion [66]. Bone scintigraphy typically demonstrates increased radionuclide uptake. The MR imaging characteristics of these tumors are non-specific with lesions generally having intermediate signal intensity on T1-weighted images and intermediate to high signal intensity on T2-weighted images (Fig. 13).

Surgical resection is often not feasible because of the lesion location and large associated soft tissue components. Chemotherapy and radiation treatment are the mainstay therapeutic options with prognosis dependent upon tumor location [65].

Osteosarcoma

Osteosarcoma of the spine is rare, accounting for 0.6% to 4% of all osteosarcomas and 5% of all primary malignant tumors of the spine [72,73]. Presentation is usually at an older age (fourth decade) than for appendicular lesions [59,73]. Similar to appendicular lesions, osteosarcoma of the spine affects more males than females. Patients often present with pain and a palpable mass and 70% to 80% have neurologic symptoms [72]. Serum alkaline phosphatase levels may be elevated due to increased bone turnover. Osteosarcomas have been reported at all levels of the spine, but appear to have a predilection for the thoracolumbar segments [73].

Spinal osteosarcomas are typically high-grade lesions. Most spinal osteosarcomas are osteoblastic in nature with the osteoid produced by the malignant cells. However, chondroblastic and fibroblastic histologic types have also been reported.

Osteosarcomas are typically better evaluated with radiographs and CT because of superior identification and characterization of the mineralized matrix (Fig. 14). Dense mineralization can give the appearance of an ivory vertebral body on radiographs or CT. Bone scintigraphy shows marked radiotracer uptake. MR imaging is useful for evaluating lesion extent, particularly in lesions with soft tissue involvement of the surrounding nerve roots and spinal canal (see Fig. 14). Lesions with abundant mineralization reveal low signal intensity on all pulse sequences.

The prognosis for patients with spinal osteosarcoma is poor despite chemotherapy and radiation treatment [72]. As with Ewing-sarcoma–PNET lesions of the spine, complete surgical resection with spinal osteosarcomas is usually not possible. Death usually occurs within 1 year of diagnosis [59].

Summary

MR imaging of the spine frequently reveals lesions that can be ascribed to degenerative changes, known metastatic disease or lymphoproliferative disease. However, in situations where solitary lesions are encountered, primary neoplasms should be considered. A multimodality approach can be used to fully characterize the lesion and the combination of information obtained from the different modalities usually narrows the diagnostic possibilities significantly. MR imaging is a particularly useful tool for providing diagnostic information and for staging the extent of the lesion in preparation for surgical resection. It is important for radiologists to be familiar with the imaging characteristics of these lesions to avoid unnecessary work-ups of benign lesions and to facilitate the treatment and management of more aggressive or malignant tumors. An overview of some of the imaging features of primary tumors of the spine is presented in Table 1.

References

[1] Murphey MD, Andrews CL, Flemming DJ, et al. From the archives of the AFIP. Primary tumors of the spine: radiologic pathologic correlation. Radiographics 1996;16:1131–58.

[2] Hall FM, Goldberg RP, Davies JA, et al. Scintigraphic assessment of bone islands. Radiology 1980;135:737–42.

[3] Azouz EM, Kozlowski K, Marton D, et al. Osteoid osteoma and osteoblastoma of the spine in children. Pediatr Radiol 1986;16:25–31.

[4] Greenspan A. Benign bone-forming lesions: osteoma, osteoid osteoma, and osteoblastoma. Skeletal Radiol 1993;22:485–500.

[5] Kransdorf MJ, Stull MA, Gilkey FW, et al. Osteoid osteoma. Radiographics 1991;11:671–96.

[6] Swank SM, Barnes RA. Osteoid osteoma in a vertebral body. Case report. Spine 1987;12:602–5.

[7] Rosenthal DI, Hornicek FJ, Torriani M, et al. Osteoid osteoma: percutaneous treatment with radiofrequency energy1. Radiology 2003;229: 171–5.

[8] Nour SG, Aschoff AJ, Mitchell ICS, et al. MR imaging-guided radio-frequency thermal ablation of the lumbar vertebrae in porcine models1. Radiology 2004;230:697–702.

[9] Gangi A, Alizadeh H, Wong L, et al. Osteoid osteoma: percutaneous laser ablation and follow-up in 114 patients. Radiology 2006;242: 293–301.

[10] Gangi A, Basile A, Buy X, et al. Radiofrequency and laser ablation of spinal lesions. Semin Ultrasound CT MR 2005;26:89–97.

[11] Kroon HM. Osteoblastoma: clinical and radiologic findings in 98 new cases. Radiology 1990; 175:783–90.

[12] Kumar R. Expansile bone lesions of the vertebra. Radiographics 1988;8:749–69.

[13] Lucas DR, Unni KK, McLeod RA, et al. Osteoblastoma: clinicopathologic study of 306 cases. Hum Pathol 1994;25:117–34.

[14] Mayer L. Malignant degeneration of so-called benign osteoblastoma. Bull Hosp Joint Dis 1967;28:4–13.

[15] Schajowicz F, Lemos C. Osteoid osteoma and osteoblastoma. Closely related entities of osteoblastic derivation. Acta Orthop Scand 1970;41: 272–91.

[16] McLeod RA, Dahlin DC, Beabout JW. The spectrum of osteoblastoma. AJR Am J Roentgenol 1976;126:321–5.

[17] Crim JR. Widespread inflammatory response to osteoblastoma: the flare phenomenon. Radiology 1990;177:835–6.

[18] Bidwell JK, Young JW, Khalluff E. Giant cell tumor of the spine: computed tomography appearance and review of the literature. J Comput Tomogr 1987;11:307–11.

[19] Schwimer SR, Bassett LW, Mancuso AA, et al. Giant cell tumor of the cervicothoracic spine. AJR Am J Roentgenol 1981;136:63–7.

[20] Smith J, Wixon D, Watson RC. Giant-cell tumor of the sacrum. Clinical and radiologic features in 13 patients. J Can Assoc Radiol 1979;30:34–9.

[21] Mirra JM, Rand F, Rand R, et al. Giant-cell tumor of the second cervical vertebra treated by cryosurgery and irradiation. Clin Orthop 1981;154:228–33.

[22] Turcotte RE, Biagini R, Sim FH, et al. Giant cell tumor of the spine and sacrum. Chir Organi Mov 1990;75:104–7.

[23] Murphey MD, Nomikos GC, Flemming DJ, et al. From the archives of AFIP. Imaging of giant cell tumor and giant cell reparative granuloma of bone: radiologic-pathologic correlation. Radiographics 2001;21:1283–309.

[24] Chhaya S, White LM, Kandel R, et al. Transarticular invasion of bone tumours across the sacroiliac joint. Skeletal Radiol 2005;34:771–7.

[25] Seider MJ, Rich TA, Ayala AG, et al. Giant cell tumors of bone: treatment with radiation therapy. Radiology 1986;161:537–40.

[26] Kransdorf MJ, Sweet DE. Aneurysmal bone cyst: concept, controversy, clinical presentation, and imaging. AJR Am J Roentgenol 1995;164:573–80.

[27] Beltran J. Aneurysmal bone cysts: MR imaging at 1.5 T. Radiology 1986;158:689–90.

[28] Mankin HJ, Hornicek FJ, Ortiz-Cruz E, et al. Aneurysmal bone cyst: a review of 150 patients. J Clin Oncol 2005;23:6756–62.

[29] Mohit AA, Eskridge J, Ellenbogen R, et al. Aneurysmal bone cyst of the atlas: successful treatment through selective arterial embolization: case report. Neurosurgery 2004;55:982.

[30] Rastogi S, Varshney MK, Trikha V, et al. Treatment of aneurysmal bone cysts with percutaneous sclerotherapy using polidocanol: a review of 72 cases with long-term follow-up. J Bone Joint Surg Br 2006;88:1212–6.

[31] Albrecht S, Crutchfield JS, SeGall GK. On spinal osteochondromas. J Neurosurg 1992;77:247–52.

[32] Fiumara E, Scarabino T, Guglielmi G, et al. Osteochondroma of the L-5 vertebra: a rare cause of sciatic pain. J Neurosurg 1999;219–22.

[33] Ratliff J, Voorhies R. Osteochondroma of the C5 lamina with cord compression: case report and review of the literature. Spine 2000;25:1293–5.

[34] Roblot P, Alcalay M, Cazenave-Roblot F, et al. Osteochondroma of the thoracic spine. Report of a case and review of the literature. Spine 1990; 15:240–3.

[35] Govender S, Parbhoo AH. Osteochondroma with compression of the spinal cord: a report of two cases. J Bone Joint Surg Br 1999;81:667–9.

[36] Palmer FJ, Blum PW. Osteochondroma with spinal cord compression: report of three cases. J Neurosurg 1980;52:842–5.

[37] Huvos AG. Hemangioma, lymphangioma, angiomatosis/lymphangiomatosis, glomus tumor. Bone tumors: diagnosis, treatment and prognosis. 2nd edition. Philadelphia: Saunders; 1991. p. 553–78.

[38] Choi JJ, Murphey MD. Angiomatous skeletal lesions. Semin Musculoskelet Radiol 2000;4: 67–74.

[39] Enzinger FM, Weiss SW. Benign tumors and tumorlike lesions of blood vessels in soft tissues tumors. St. Louis (MO): Mosby-Year Book; 1995. p. 579–26.

[40] Laredo JD. Vertebral hemangiomas: fat content as a sign of aggressiveness. Radiology 1990; 177:467–72.

[41] Acosta FL Jr, Dowd CF, Chin C, et al. Current treatment strategies and outcomes in the management of symptomatic vertebral hemangiomas. Neurosurgery 2006;58:287–95.

[42] Fox MW, Onofrio BM. The natural history and management of symptomatic and asymptomatic vertebral hemangiomas. J Neurosurg 1993;78: 36–45.

[43] Friedman DP. Symptomatic vertebral hemangiomas: MR findings. AJR Am J Roentgenol 1996; 167:359–64.

[44] Kransdorf MJ, Smith SE. Lesions of unknown histogenesis: langerhans cell histiocytosis and ewingsarcoma. Semin Musculoskelet Radiol 2000;4:75–86.

[45] Nesbit ME, Kieffer S, D'Angio GJ. Reconstitution of vertebral height in histiocytosis X: a long-term follow-up. J Bone Joint Surg 1969;51:1360–8.

[46] Stull MA. Langerhans cell histiocytosis of bone. RadioGraphics 1992;12:801–23.

[47] Brown CW, Jarvis JG, Letts M, et al. Treatment and outcome of vertebral langerhans cell histiocytosis at the Children's Hospital of Eastern Ontario. Can J Surg 2005;48:230–6.

[48] Kaplan GR, Saifuddin A, Pringle JA, et al. Langerhans' cell histiocytosis of the spine: use of MRI in guiding biopsy. Skeletal Radiol 1998; 27:673–6.

[49] Bianchi PM, Marsella P, Masi R, et al. Cervical chordoma in childhood: clinical statistical contribution. Int J Pediatr Otorhinolaryngol 1989; 18:39–45.

[50] Eriksson B, Gunterberg B, Kindblom LG. Chordoma. A clinicopathologic and prognostic study of a Swedish national series. Acta Orthop Scand 1981;52:49–58.

[51] Healey JH, Lane JM. Chordoma: a critical review of diagnosis and treatment. Orthop Clin North Am 1989;20:417–26.

[52] Sundaresan N, Galicich JH, Chu FC, et al. Spinal chordomas. J Neurosurg 1979;50:312–9.

[53] Wippold FJ, Koeller KK, Smirniotopoulos JG. Clinical and imaging features of cervical chordoma. AJR Am J Roentgenol 1999;172:1423–6.

[54] de Bruine FT, Kroon HM. Spinal chordoma: radiologic features in 14 cases. AJR Am J Roentgenol 1988;150:861–3.

[55] Sung MS, Lee GK, Kang HS, et al. Sacrococcygeal chordoma: MR imaging in 30 patients. Skeletal Radiol 2005;34:87–94.

[56] Firooznia H, Golimbu C, Rafii M, et al. Computed tomography of spinal chordomas. J Comput Tomogr 1986;10:45–50.

[57] Firooznia H, Pinto RS, Lin JP, et al. Chordoma: radiologic evaluation of 20 cases. AJR Am J Roentgenol 1976;127:797–805.

[58] Rosenthal DI, Scott JA, Mankin HJ, et al. Sacrococcygeal chordoma: magnetic resonance imaging and computed tomography. AJR Am J Roentgenol 1985;145:143–7.

[59] Flemming DJ, Murphey MD, Carmichael BB, et al. Primary tumors of the spine. Semin Musculoskelet Radiol 2000;4:2–208.

[60] Hirsh LF, Thanki A, Spector HB. Primary spinal chondrosarcoma with eighteen-year follow-up: case report and literature review. Case reports. Neurosurgery 1984;14:747–9.

[61] Shives TC, McLeod RA, Unni KK, et al. Chondrosarcoma of the spine. J Bone Joint Surg 1989;71: 1158–65.

[62] Subbarao K, Jacobson HG. Primary malignant neoplasms. Semin Roentgenol 1979;14:44–57.

[63] Grubb MR, Currier BL, Pritchard DJ, et al. Primary Ewing's sarcoma of the spine. Spine 1994;19:309–13.

[64] Pilepich MV, Vietti TJ, Nesbit ME, et al. Ewing's sarcoma of the vertebral column. Int J Radiat Oncol Biol Phys 1981;7:27–31.

[65] Sharafuddin MJ, Haddad FS, Hitchon PW, et al. Treatment options in primary Ewing's sarcoma of the spine: report of seven cases and review of the literature. Neurosurgery 1992;30:610–8.

[66] Ilaslan H, Sundaram M, Unni KK, et al. Primary Ewing's sarcoma of the vertebral column. Skeletal Radiol 2004;33:506–13.

[67] Drevelegas A, Chourmouzi D, Boulogianni G, et al. Imaging of primary bone tumors of the spine. Eur Radiol 2003;13:1859–71.

[68] Shirley SK, Gilula LA, Siegal GP, et al. Roentgenographic-pathologic correlation of diffuse sclerosis in Ewing sarcoma of bone. Skeletal Radiol 1984;12:69–78.

[69] Kornberg M. Primary Ewing's sarcoma of the spine. A review and case report. Spine 1986;11:54–7.

[70] Mohan V, Sabri T, Gupta RP, et al. Solitary ivory vertebra due to primary Ewing's sarcoma. Pediatr Radiol 1992;22:388–90.

[71] Weinstein JB, Siegel MJ, Griffith RC. Spinal Ewing sarcoma: misleading appearances. Skeletal Radiol 1984;11:262–5.

[72] Barwick KW, Huvos AG, Smith J. Primary osteogenic sarcoma of the vertebral column: a clinicopathologic correlation of ten patients. Cancer 1980;46:595–604.

[73] Ilaslan H, Sundaram M, Unni KK, et al. Primary vertebral osteosarcoma: imaging findings 1. RSNA; 2004.

MAGNETIC
RESONANCE
IMAGING CLINICS

Magn Reson Imaging Clin N Am 15 (2007) 257–271

MR Imaging and Osseous Spinal Intervention and Intervertebral Disk Intervention

Rick W. Obray, MD[a],*, Ross W. Filice, MD[a], Douglas P. Beall, MD[b,c]

- MR imaging and osseous spinal intervention
  Vertebroplasty
  Kyphoplasty
  Spineoplasty
- MR imaging of intervertebral disk intervention

Percutaneous disk decompression
Percutaneous rhizotomy
- General complications
- Summary
- References

Back pain is one of the most common ailments in the United States, second only to headache in terms of the number of annual physician visits [1,2]. Back pain has multiple etiologies and can originate in various anatomic regions of the spine: the osseous portions, the joints, the muscles, the nerves, and the intervertebral disks. Until recently, treatment for persistent, severe back pain deemed refractory to conservative therapy often ultimately resulted in open surgery. Percutaneous spine intervention, a wide range of invasive spine procedures performed through a puncture hole or through a small incision not requiring soft tissue closure and with few or no skin sutures or staples, is rapidly emerging as an effective alternative to open surgery. Such interventions are expanding dramatically in terms of both the number and types of procedures performed.

Because of the large number of people with back pain requiring more advanced therapy and because

of the potential advantages of minimally invasive therapy, this area has tremendous growth potential [3,4]. The modern diagnostic radiologist must acquire a general understanding of the procedures being performed, the postprocedural MR imaging appearance of the spine, and the complications that may arise.

In this article, the authors describe many of the minimally invasive osseous, intervertebral disk, and spinal nerve interventions currently being performed. Some of these procedures have been performed for longer periods and are more widely established. Others have been developed more recently and are less widely performed. A general introduction to these types of procedures is provided, along with the characteristic pre- and postprocedural MR imaging appearance related to these techniques. Reported and theoretical complications that may arise and their respective MR imaging appearances are also be discussed.

a Department of Radiology, Johns Hopkins Hospital, 600 North Wolfe Street, Baltimore, MD 21283, USA
b Clinical Radiology of Oklahoma, P.O. Box 721688, Oklahoma City, OK 73172-1688, USA
c University of Oklahoma, 610 NW 14th Street, Oklahoma City, OK 73103, USA
* Corresponding author.
E-mail address: robray1@jhmi.edu (R.W. Obray).

mri.theclinics.com

doi:10.1016/j.mric.2007.05.001

MR imaging and osseous spinal intervention

Osseous spinal interventions for the treatment of pain related to vertebral compression fractures have increased dramatically since vertebroplasty was first introduced in the literature by Galibert and colleagues in 1987 [5]. These techniques include vertebroplasty and kyphoplasty, as well as newer techniques, such as spineoplasty and arcuplasty. The growing popularity of these types of procedures is understandable given that over 700,000 vertebral compression fractures occur in the United States each year [6,7], and that vertebroplasty and kyphoplasty have been demonstrated to be safe and effective interventions [8–12]. This section briefly presents the types of osseous spinal interventions currently being performed, the potential complications associated with them, and their postprocedural MR imaging appearance.

Vertebroplasty

Vertebroplasty is a percutaneous, image-guided procedure performed for the treatment of pain associated with compression fractures related to osteoporosis, malignancy, or hemangiomas [8–17]. It involves the percutaneous placement of bone cement into fractured vertebral bodies through a needle placed via a transpedicular or a parapedicular approach [8,18]. It is generally well tolerated and may be performed as an outpatient procedure. The procedure usually takes approximately 15 to 45 minutes per vertebral level, and the time necessary to perform the vertebroplasty mostly depends on the severity of the fracture.

Vertebral bodies treated with vertebroplasty have a distinctive appearance on MR imaging, although there is some variability depending on the type of bone cement used. Polymethylmethacrylate (PMMA), the chemical name for bone cement, is the most common material used, and it appears hyperdense on CT and dark on all standard MR imaging pulse sequences (Fig. 1).

No one has determined what amount of cement is best for pain relief and that issue remains controversial. Generally, a uniform filling of 50% to 75% of the vertebral body is desired, and care should be taken to prevent cement extravasation. Injecting higher cement volumes has not been demonstrated to provide increased pain relief, and injecting a large amount of cement may increase the stiffness of the fractured vertebral level more than that of its prefracture level. In an ex vivo study, Belkoff and colleagues [19] performed bilateral injections of bone cement into fractured osteoporotic vertebral bodies and found that as little as 2 mL of cement was enough to restore preinjury strength, but a total of 4 to 8 mL was necessary to restore preinjury stiffness, depending on the type of cement and the vertebral body level treated. Kosmopoulos and colleagues [20] found that restoration of stiffness with vertebroplasty is best attained with 3 to 5 mL of cement properly placed in the central portion of the vertebral body, but that complete replacement of the marrow volume resulted in an apparent stiffness above preinjury.

Also, the individual interpreting MR imaging of the spine should be aware of the importance of cement placement within the vertebral body. Dean and colleagues [21] evaluated the concept that cement placement is more important than injected volume or percentage of filled vertebral body. The investigators found an asymmetric flow pattern of cement when using a standard unilateral vertebroplasty technique to inject cadaveric vertebral bodies. The strength of the injected vertebral bodies was greater than that of the noninjected control group. However, the magnitude of strength increase did not correlate with the amount of cement

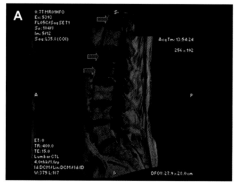
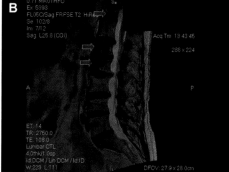

Fig. 1. (*A, B*) Sagittal T2-weighted MR imaging of lower thoracic and lumbar spine following treatment of T11, L1, and L2 vertebroplasty with PMMA. Bone cement appears dark on all sequences (*arrows*).

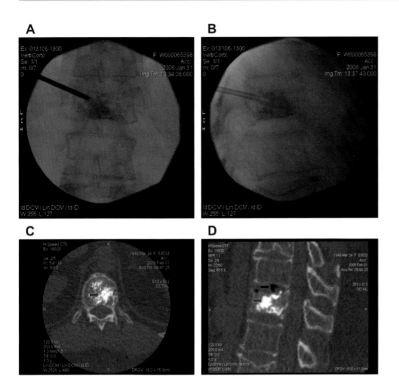

Fig. 2. Views of T12 vertebral body following vertebroplasty with synthetic cortical bone cement. The synthetic cortical bone cement appears slightly less dense than PMMA. (*A*) Anterio-posterior view. (*B*) Lateral view. (*C*) Axial CT. Arrow points to synthetic cortical bone cement. (*D*) Sagittal CT. Blue arrow points to synthetic cortical bone cement. Air is seen within the disc space (*black arrow*).

injected. They suggested that a well-placed column between the endplates may be more important to strengthening the vertebral body than simply stiffening the trabecular matrix with cement.

Several experimental bone cements (or resin polymers) are currently being developed but have not as yet gained widespread use. One, advertised as synthetic bone cement, is a polymer-reinforced composite that is less dense that PMMA (Fig. 2). It was designed to have mechanical properties more similar than PMMA to bone. Given this likeness, the hope for this material is that it will link to medullary bone with an interface that does not involve a border of fibrous tissue and that its biomechanical similarities to cortical bone will reduce the occurrence of adjacent level fractures. This synthetic cortical bone also appears hyperdense on CT, although less dense than PMMA, and dark on all standard pulse sequences (Fig. 3).

Major reported complications related to vertebroplasty are uncommon, especially when the procedure is performed by experienced interventional radiologists. The complications that are seen may be divided into those that arise from

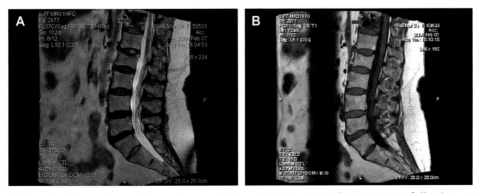

Fig. 3. (*A*) Sagittal T1-weighted MR imaging and (*B*) sagittal T2-weighted MR imaging following successful vertebroplasty of T12 vertebral body with synthetic cortical bone cement. Although less dense than PMMA, injected cement still appears dark on all standard MR imaging sequences (*arrows*).

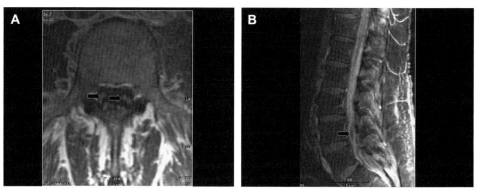

Fig. 4. Complications following vertebroplasty. (*A*) Axial T1-weighted MR imaging and (*B*) sagittal T2-weighted MR imaging following PMMA midthoracic spine vertebroplasty (treated level not shown) demonstrating clumping and enhancement of the lower lumbar and sacral nerve roots within the thecal sac (*arrows*), compatible with arachnoiditis.

the injection of bone cement into the vertebral body and those that arise as a result of gaining access to the vertebral body [22,23]. Complications related to gaining access to the vertebral body include bleeding, infection, fracture of the pedicle, puncture of the dura with development of arachnoiditis, and neurologic injury (Fig. 4). Complications related to cement injection include neurologic injury either from transforaminal or epidural cement extravasation, pulmonary embolus, allergic reaction, and fracture of adjacent vertebral bodies (Fig. 5).

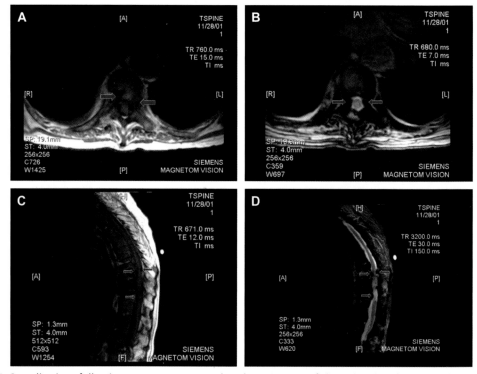

Fig. 5. Complications following percutaneous vertebroplasty. Images of thoracic spine demonstrating epidural extravasation of PMMA immediately following percutaneous vertebroplasty. (*A*) Axial T1-weighted image. (*B*) Axial T2-weighted image. (*C*) Sagittal T1-weighted image. (*D*) Sagittal T2-weighted image. PMMA appears as dark signal in the epidural space on both T1- and T2-weighted sequences (*arrows*).

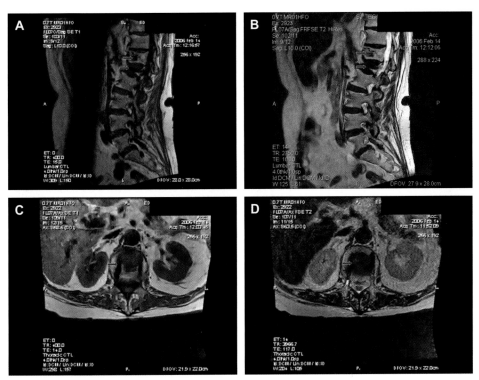

Fig. 6. Images of thoracic spine following successful treatment of vertebral plana with kyphoplasty. (*A*) Sagittal T1-weighted MR imaging. (*B*) Sagittal T2-weighted MR imaging. (*C*) Axial T1-weighted MR imaging. (*D*) Axial T2-weighted MR imaging. Like cement used in vertebroplasty, kyphoplasty cement is dark (*arrows* in *C* and *D*) on all standard pulse sequences. Patient reported excellent pain control following the procedure.

Kyphoplasty

Kyphoplasty is another osseous spinal intervention performed for the treatment of pain associated with vertebral compression fractures. Kyphoplasty, developed in the early 1990s by an orthopedic surgeon, uses balloons to reduce vertebral compression fractures before the injection of PMMA. This technique also uses needles that are placed using a parapedicular or transpedicular approach and is, essentially, a derivation of vertebroplasty [24,25]. Like vertebroplasty, kyphoplasty involves the percutaneous injection of bone cement through a needle. However, unlike vertebroplasty, kyphoplasty uses a drill and inflatable balloons designed to reduce the

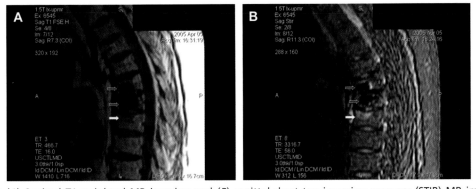

Fig. 7. (*A*) Sagittal T1-weighted MR imaging and (*B*) sagittal short tau inversion recovery (STIR) MR imaging following remote percutaneous kyphoplasty of two adjacent vertebral bodies (*blue arrows*), demonstrating decreased marrow signal on T1-weighted images and increased signal on STIR images within vertebral body inferior to lower treated level (*white arrows*), compatible with edema related to acute fracture.

fracture and to create a cavity before cement injection. It has been reported that the kyphotic deformity related to the compression fracture increases morbidity and mortality due to reduced pulmonary function, early satiety, decreased mobility, and decreased quality of life [22,26–29]. It has also been reported that the creation of an intraosseous cavity may decrease the risk of cement extravasation during injection [30]. The decreased extravasation and the increased fracture reduction achieved using kyphoplasty are both controversial and are currently being debated in the literature [12,29–31].

On MR imaging, the vertebral bodies treated with kyphoplasty appear dark on all standard sequences (Fig. 6). Because of the cavity created before cement injection, the injected cement tends to be more localized near the site of injection within the vertebral body when compared with fractures treated with vertebroplasty (see Fig. 3).

Complications associated with kyphoplasty [23] are similar to those observed with vertebroplasty and include bleeding and epidural hematoma; infection; neurologic injury from direct trauma related to needle placement, transforaminal cement extravasation, or epidural cement extravasation; pulmonary embolus; dural puncture; fracture of the pedicle; and fractures of the adjacent vertebral bodies (Fig. 7).

Spineoplasty

A new vertebral augmentation technique known as spineoplasty is a percutaneous spinal intervention that involves the placement of allograft bone into a mesh implant that is placed within a fractured vertebral body [32]. Although spineoplasty is similar to vertebroplasty and kyphoplasty in that all are methods to treat vertebral compression fractures, there are some key differences. First, the working access to the vertebral body in spineoplasty is attained with a larger-caliber system than that for either vertebroplasty or kyphoplasty and requires a parapedicular approach to the vertebral body. This larger-caliber system is needed for using the surgical instruments that remodel or core the interior of the vertebral body before the placement of particulate allograft bone material [33]. The

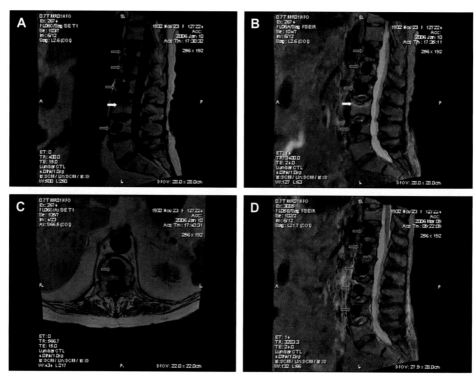

Fig. 8. Images of lumbar spine status postspinoplasty. Sagittal (*A, B*) and axial (*C*) T1-weighted MR imaging at L1, L2, L3, and L5. Images show allograft bone material (dark on all sequences (*blue arrows*)) within mesh within treated vertebral bodies. Adjacent level vertebral fracture is noted at L4, as evidence by decreased signal on sagittal T1-weighted sequence (*white arrow* in *A*) and increased signal on sagittal T2-weighted sequence (*white arrow* in *B*). (*D*) Sagittal T1-weighted MR imaging postspinoplasty at L1 through L5. Adjacent level vertebral fracture at L4 (*white arrows* in *A* and *B*) has now been treated (*blue arrow* at L4 in *D*).

procedure is generally well tolerated and can be performed as an outpatient or inpatient procedure, depending on the patient's health.

The immediate post procedural magnetic resonance appearance of vertebral compression fractures treated via spineoplasty is similar to that of vertebroplasty and kyphoplasty in that the allograft bone is dark on all pulse sequences (Fig. 8). The appearance differs from that of PMMA in that the allograft bone pack appears as a well-defined elliptical implant that does not extend into the interstices of the cancellous bone.

Potential complications related to spineoplasty can be divided into those associated with placement of the needle/coaxial system and those related to injection of the allograft bone. Because of the large caliber of the coaxial system and the parapedicular approach used with spineoplasty, the theoretical risk of paraspinal or epidural bleeding as well as potential traumatic damage to the exiting spinal nerve roots may be increased with this technique as compared with kyphoplasty or vertebroplasty. Like vertebroplasty and kyphoplasty, fracture of the adjacent vertebral bodies can also be seen with spineoplasty (see Fig. 8) but an early

hope for the procedure is a lesser rate of adjacent level fracture due to the similarity of the biomechanical properties of the bone graft implant relative to that of the adjacent vertebral bodies. The risk of extravasation of the material placed into the vertebral body decreases with the containment provided by the mesh implant but is not altogether eliminated (Fig. 9).

MR imaging of intervertebral disk intervention

Percutaneous disk decompression

Disk herniation is a prevalent etiology of back pain and neurogenic pain in adults [2] but disk herniations can also be seen in adolescents and even children [34–36]. Approximately 200,000 lumbar disk procedures are performed annually in the United States [37]. Medical costs related to back pain are measured in the billions of dollars [38,39]. The traditional approach to disk herniation has been to initially treat conservatively with medication, rest, and activity modification. If conservative therapy fails, surgical intervention typically follows with a discectomy and/or a partial laminectomy

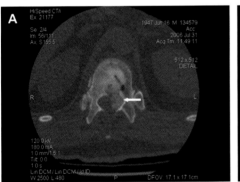
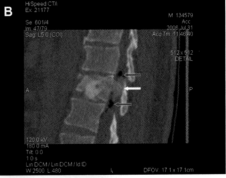
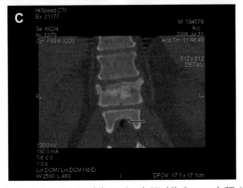

Fig. 9. Images following spineoplasty. (*A*) Axial CT. (*B*) Sagittal CT. (*C*) Coronol CT. Images demonstrate rupture of the mesh allograft bone container and extravasation of the bone graft (*white arrows* in *A* and *B*) and air (*blue arrows* in *B* and *C*) into the epidural space. Surprisingly the patient exhibited no significant clinical syndromes associated with the allograft extravasation.

as common treatments of choice. More invasive treatment is typically initiated when a progressive motor, sensory, or reflex change is noted on serial neurologic examinations. In this clinical scenario, surgical disk decompression has produced clinical improvements by decreasing the size of the intervertebral disk herniation; thereby decreasing the pressure on the adjacent nerve root [40]. Because some patients do not respond well to conventional surgical techniques [41] and because of the complications associated with open surgery [35,36, 42–46], alternative therapies have been developed. One primary alternative to open surgery is percutaneous disk decompression. The objective of percutaneous decompression, similar to that of open surgery, is to relieve pressure within the intervertebral disk. This decreased intradiscal pressure may result in decreased pressure against the adjacent nerve root and decreased neurogenic pain [35,36, 46–48]. At one time, this could only be accomplished by manual removal of the disk contents [49]. Over time, however, other methods have been developed, including automated nucleus removal [35,36,46,50] and destruction of the nucleus

with either chemicals [48,51], heat [52,53], or laser therapy [54]. Percutaneous disk decompression has been shown to be a safe procedure with a low rate of complications. Furthermore, percutaneous disk decompression has proven effective at treating back and neurogenic pain related to disk herniation [35,36,46,50–56].

In percutaneous disk decompression, a cannula is introduced to the level of the intervertebral disk via an oblique approach that enters the disk just anterior to the superior articular process (an approach that is identical to that used for standard discography). Next, a needle is inserted through the cannula and an incision is made through the annulus of the intervertebral disk. The needle is then advanced into the nucleus pulposis. Once the cannula is placed, iodinated contrast material may be injected to visualize the posterolateral nuclear–annular border. A depth stop is then positioned on the cannula to mark this boundary and a titanium auger device is inserted through the cannula. The auger is attached to a disposable rotary motor, which mechanically aspirates nuclear material proximally into a chamber on the distal portion of the rotary

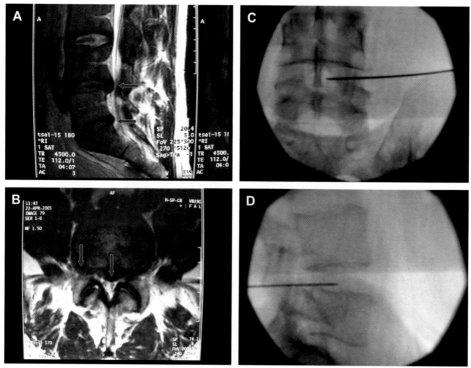

Fig. 10. (A) Sagittal T2-weighted and (B) axial T2-weighted preintervention MR imaging of the lumbar spine demonstrating a broad-based disk protrusion (*arrows*) with bilateral facet hypertrophy at L4-5 causing bilateral neural foraminal and thecal sac narrowing. A smaller posterior disk protrusion is seen at L5-S1. (C) Anteroposterior and (D) lateral fluoroscopic spot images obtained during percutaneous disk decompression with proper localization of the tip of the decompression cannula within the L4-L5 disk space.

motor device. Typically, the herniation is decompressed for an average of 3 minutes and between 0.5 to 2 mL of disk material is removed. The goal, as described above, is to relieve pressure within the disk so that the posterior protrusion or extrusion will be decompressed; thereby decreasing the size of the herniation and relieving pressure on the spinal cord and/or nerve root [57,58].

The primary complications that may arise include infection and hematoma, but there is also a potential for neurological complications, including injury to the dorsal or ventral rami. There are also other theoretical complications when performing the procedure in the thoracic or cervical spine, including pleural tearing, pneumothorax, and injury to the recurrent laryngeal nerve.

Imaging after percutaneous disk decompression may not change dramatically from imaging before intervention. Often, the disk bulge or protrusion will look slightly smaller, but the change can be minimal. The actual intervention itself does not cause any changes that are visible on CT or MR imaging (Figs. 10–12). Success of the procedure is generally determined from a clinical and symptomatic perspective.

Percutaneous rhizotomy

Facet joint pain is another large contributor to chronic back pain [59–61]. Degenerative changes of the facet joints can cause pain from the arthritic change itself or may cause irritation of the medial branches of the dorsal rami, giving rise to chronic neurogenic pain. If the facet pain is refractory to conservative treatment, facet joint injections with local anesthetic and steroids are typically performed [59,62,63]. If these injections confirm the location and source of the pain, but are not effective in providing long-term pain relief, ablation or transection of the medial branch of the dorsal ramus is an alternative. A procedure known as a rhizotomy involves the percutaneous ablation of the medial branch of the dorsal ramus and can be advantageous because of the minimally invasive nature of the procedure and the low rate of complications [64].

The goal in percutaneous rhizotomy is to destroy the afferent nerve supply to the facet joints. A radioablation probe is introduced at the level of the target nerve root via a paramedian approach, and the tip of the probe is placed parallel to the target nerve in the notch at the junction between the ipsilateral

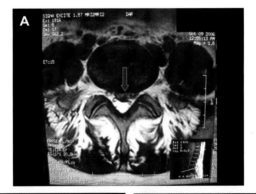

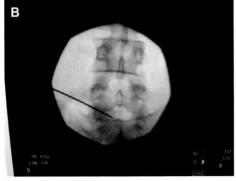
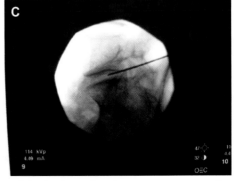

Fig. 11. (A) Axial T2-weighted preintervention MR image of the lumbar spine demonstrates a central posterior disk protrusion at L5-S1 (*blue arrow*) causing narrowing of the left neural foramen at that level. (B) Anteroposterior and (C) lateral fluoroscopic spot image obtained during percutaneous disk decompression demonstrates proper localization of the decompression cannula within the L5-S1 disk space.

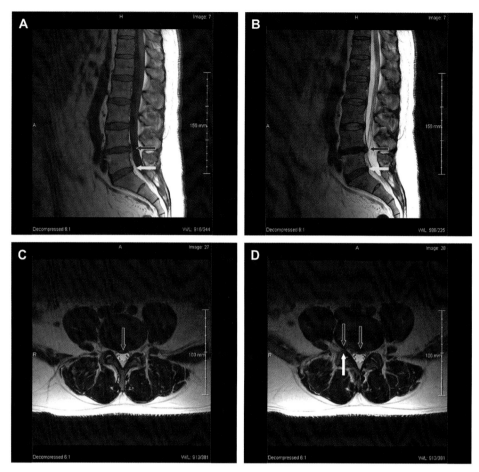

Fig. 12. Preintervention MR images of the lumbar spine. (*A*) Sagittal T1-weighted MR image. (*B*) Sagittal T2-weighted MR image. (*C, D*) Axial T2-weighted MR images. Images demonstrate a central and right foraminal disk protrusion (*blue arrows*) as well as facet hypertrophy causing narrowing of the right neural foramen (*white arrow*) and the thecal sac. A smaller posterior disk protrusion is also seen at L5-S1 (*yellow arrow*). Because the patient was experiencing significant symptoms, percutaneous disk decompression was performed at the L4-L5 level. (*E*) Sagittal T1-weighted, (*F*) sagittal T2-weighted, and (*G, H*) axial T2-weighted postintervention MR images of the lumbar spine demonstrate only a slight decrease in the size of the disk protrusions (*blue arrows*) and persistent narrowing of the right neural foramen at L4-5 (*white arrow* in *H*). Yellow arrows (in *E* and *F*) point to a small disc protrusion postprocedurally. Despite the lack of significant anatomic changes, the patient's symptoms had dramatically improved.

transverse process and the superior articular process. The target nerve root can be tested by applying low-voltage current while the patient is under mild conscious sedation to ensure correct placement. Alternating current is then applied through the probe, generally at 500 kilocycles per second. As current flows through the tissues surrounding the probe, the resistance of the tissues causes heating. Early cytotoxic response occurs at 50°C, but temperatures of 70°C to 80°C should be attained for the best chance of permanent ablation. Radiofrequency ablation should be performed for 60 to 90 seconds. The zone of tissue destruction is an elliptical shape of approximately one to 1.5 times the diameter of

the probe. Different probe sizes are available including 18-, 20-, and 22-gauge probes. Larger probes such as the 18-gauge probe should be used in the lumbar spine for best results, while smaller probes can be used in the cervical spine. If there is incomplete destruction of the target nerve, regeneration can occur in 9 to 12 months. Radiofrequency ablation is associated with low morbidity and can easily be performed again on the same nerve [65,66].

As with any percutaneous intervention, complications that may arise include infection and hematoma, as well as injury to the lung or pleura with thoracic interventions. Complications specifically

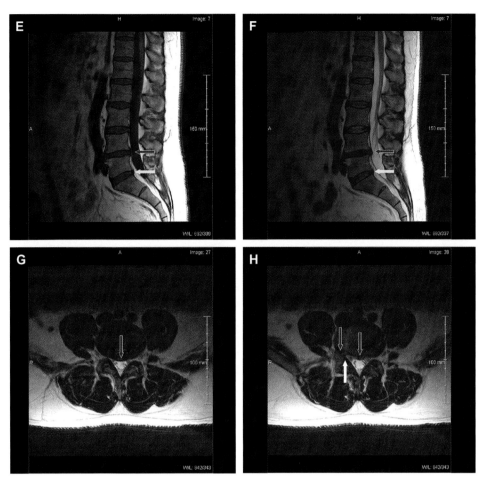

Fig. 12 continued

related to rhizotomy may also occur, such as injury to the surrounding nerves, including the ventral ramus or other branches of the dorsal ramus (intermediate or lateral branches).

Imaging is not routinely performed before or after percutaneous rhizotomy, primarily because of the limits of contrast and spatial resolution of CT and MR imaging. This limitation does not allow consistent visualization of the dorsal nerves. If cross-sectional imaging is performed, however, fatty changes are sometimes seen in the multifidus related to postrhizotomy denervation (Fig. 13).

General complications

In general, complications that can be seen after any percutaneous intervention in the spine include bleeding, thecal sac injury, infection, and nerve injury. The blood vessels most at risk for traumatic injury during percutaneous spine intervention are the segmental arteries and veins. The most dangerous type of hemorrhage is an epidural hematoma, which can compress the spinal cord or cauda equina (Fig. 14). Less critically located hematomas can also be seen in the surrounding paravertebral musculature and subcutaneous soft tissues. Another major potential complication is infection. This is most severe when it occurs within the thecal sac. Infection and inflammation can involve the spinal cord and nerve roots, and abscesses can also form, especially in the epidural space. Theoretically, infection within the thecal sac could also extend rostrally and cause meningitis. Other possible infection-related complications include abscess formation in the paravertebral musculature and in the subcutaneous soft tissues. Discitis or spondylodiscitis may also occur, particularly after percutaneous disk intervention. The ventral and dorsal nerve roots are at risk for accidental injury during many of the percutaneous spine interventions. Routine CT and MR imaging do not have adequate resolution to demonstrate nerve injuries in this location,

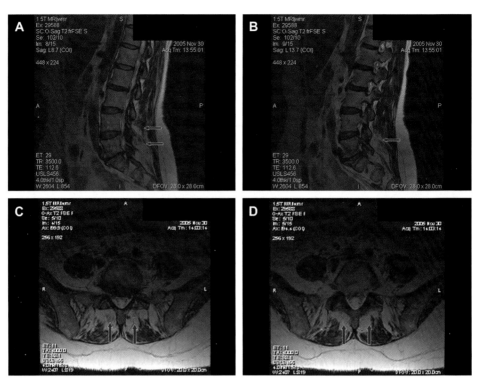

Fig. 13. Images demonstrating atrophy of the paravertebral musculature with fatty change at the level of a prior rhizotomy (*arrows*). (*A, B*) Sagittal T2-weighted MR images. (*C, D*) Axial T2-weighted MR images. This fatty atrophy of the musculature is a normal postrhizotomy finding related to denervation.

and these injuries are therefore typically established clinically.

Summary

Back pain is a major cause of morbidity and mortality in the United States. The number of percutaneous spine interventions developed to treat back

pain has dramatically increased and will likely continue to increase given the prevalence of back pain and the invasiveness of many of the current treatment regimens. The radiologist can play a central role in the implementation and development of these types of procedures by acquiring familiarity with them. An understanding of the typical pre- and postprocedural MR imaging appearance of

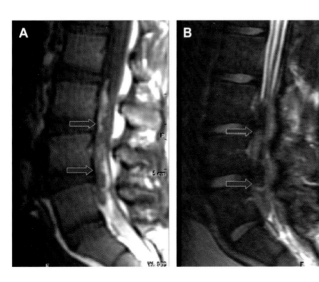

Fig. 14. (*A*) Sagittal T1-weighted and (*B*) sagittal T2-weighted MR images of the lumbar spine demonstrate an epidural hematoma surrounding the thecal sac at the L3-L5 levels (*arrows*).

percutaneous spine interventions and the appearance of the most common complications is also important for the appropriate management of patients who have undergone these procedures.

References

[1] National Institute of Neurological Disorders and Stroke. Back pain information page-Available at: http://www.ninds.nih.gov/disorders/backpain/backpain.htm. Accessed June 2006.

[2] Manek NJ, MacGregor AJ. Epidemiology of back disorders: prevalence, risk factors, and prognosis. Curr Opin Rheumatol 2005;17(2):134–40.

[3] Fessler RG, O'Toole JE, Eichholz KM, et al. The development of minimally invasive spine surgery. Neurosurg Clin N Am 2006;17(4):401–9.

[4] Kelekis AD, Somon T, Yilmaz H, et al. Interventional spine procedures. Eur J Radiol 2005; 55(3):362–83.

[5] Galibert P, Deramond H, Rosat P, et al. [Preliminary note on the treatment of vertebral angioma by percutaneous acrylic vertebroplasty]. Neurochirurgie 1987;33:166–8 [in French].

[6] National Osteoporosis Foundation. 2003 annual report. Available at: www.nof.org/news/2003-final-ar-pdf. Accessed June 2006.

[7] Melton LJ, Chrischilles EA, Cooper C, et al. How many women have osteoporosis? JBMR anniversary classic. J Bone Miner Res 2005;20(5): 886–92.

[8] Kallmes D, Jensen ME. Percutaneous vertebroplasty [review]. Radiology 2003;229(1):27–36.

[9] Mathis JM, Barr JD, Belkoff SM, et al. Percutaneous vertebroplasty: a developing standard of care for vertebral compression fractures. AJNR Am J Neuroradiol 2000;21(10):1807–12.

[10] Murphy KJ, Deramond H. Percutaneous vertebroplasty in benign and malignant disease [review]. Neuroimaging Clin N Am 2000;10(3): 535–45.

[11] Hammond A, Riley LH 3rd, Gailloud P, et al. Treatment consideration for vertebroplasty in men. AJNR Am J Neuroradiol 2004;25(4): 639–41.

[12] Evan AJ, Jensen ME, Kip KE, et al. Vertebral compression fractures: pain reduction and improvement in functional mobility after percutaneous polymethylmethacrylate vertebroplasty—retrospective report of 245 cases. Radiology 2003; 226(2):366–72.

[13] Brown DB, Gilula LA, Sehgal M, et al. Treatment of chronic symptomatic vertebral compression fractures with percutaneous vertebroplasty. AJR Am J Neuroradiol 2004;182:319–22.

[14] Zoarski GH, Snow P, Olan WJ, et al. Percutaneous vertebroplasty for osteoporotic compression fractures: quantitative prospective evaluation of long-term outcomes. J Vasc Interv Radiol 2002; 13:139–48.

[15] Weill A, Chiras J, Simon JM, et al. Spinal metastases: indications for and results of percutaneous injection of acrylic surgical cement. Radiology 1996;199:241–7.

[16] Barr JD, Barr MS, Lemley TJ, et al. Percutaneous vertebroplasty for pain relief and spinal stabilization. Spine 2000;25:923–8.

[17] Jensen ME, Evans AJ, Mathis JM, et al. Percutaneous polymethylmethacrylate vertebroplasty in the treatment of osteoporotic vertebral body compression fractures: technical aspects. AJNR Am J Neuroradiol 1997;18:1897–904.

[18] Beall DP, Braswell JJ, Martin HD, et al. Technical strategies and anatomic considerations for parapedicular access to thoracic and lumbar vertebral bodies. Skeletal Radiol 2007;36:47–52.

[19] Belkoff SM, Mathis JM, Jasper LE, et al. The biomechanics of vertebroplasty: the effect of cement volume on mechanical behavior. Spine 2001;26: 1537–41.

[20] Kosmopoulos V, Keller TS, Liebschner MAK. Finite element modeling of vertebral damage and repair. Presented at the 10th Annual Symposium on Computational Methods in Orthopaedic Biomechanics, University of Texas Southwestern Medical Center, Dallas (TX), February 9, 2002.

[21] Dean JR, Ison KT, Gishen P. The strengthening effect of percutaneous vertebroplasty. Clin Radiol 2000;55:471–6.

[22] Laredo JD, Hamze B. Complications of percutaneous vertebroplasty and their prevention. Skeletal Radiol 2004;33:493–505.

[23] David A, Nussbaum, Philippe Gailloud, Murphy Kieran. A review of complications associated with vertebroplasty and kyphoplasty as reported to the Food and Drug Administration medical device related Web site. J Vasc Interv Radiol 2004;15:1185–92.

[24] Lieberman IH, Dudeney S, Reinhardt M-K, et al. Initial outcome and efficacy of "kyphoplasty" in the treatment of painful osteoporotic vertebral compression fractures. Spine 2001;26:1631–8.

[25] Ledlie J, Renfroe M. Balloon kyphoplasty: one year outcomes in vertebral body height restoration, chronic pain, and activity levels. J Neurosurg 2003;98:36–42.

[26] Lombardi I, Oliveira LM, Mayer AF, et al. Evaluation of pulmonary function and quality of life in women with osteoporosis. Osteoporos Int 2005;16(10):1247–53 [Epub 2005 Apr 2].

[27] Culham EG, Jimenez HA, King CE, et al. Thoracic kyphosis, rib mobility, and lung volumes in normal women and women with osteoporosis. Spine 1994;19(11):1250–5.

[28] Silverman SL. The osteoporosis questionaire (OPAQ): a reliable and valid disease-targeted measure of health related quality of life in osteoporosis. Qual Life Res 2000;9:767–74.

[29] Grados F, Depriester C, Cayrolle G, et al. Long-term observations of vertebral osteoporotic fractures treated by percutaneous vertebroplasty. Rheumatology (Oxford) 2000;39:1410–4.

[30] Phillips FM, Todd Wetzel F, Lieberman I, et al. An in vivo comparison of the potential for extravertebral cement leak after vertebroplasty and kyphoplasty. Spine 2002;27(19):2173–9.

[31] Cortet B, Cotten A, Boutry N, et al. Percutaneous vertebroplasty in the treatment of osteoporotic vertebral compression fractures: an open prospective study. J Rheumatol 1999;26: 2222–8.

[32] Kuslich SD. Toward a safer method of vertebroplasty: elevation and stabilization of vertebral compression fractures with a novel, inflatable, implantable, minimally porous mesh container. In: Szpalski M, Gunzburg R, editors. Vertebral osteoporotic compression fractures. Philadelphia: Lippincott; 2003. p. 199–210.

[33] Schultz K, Stewart T, Chandler G, et al. Early experience with a minimally invasive vertebral reconstruction technique utilizing contained bone graft. Presented at the American Association of Neurological Surgeons/Congress of Neurological Surgeons. Phoenix (AZ), February 16–19, 2003.

[34] Frino J, McCarthy RE, Sparks CY, et al. Trends in adolescent lumbar disk herniation. J Pediatr Orthop 2006;26(5):579–81.

[35] Alo KM, Wright RE, Sutcliffe J, et al. Percutaneous lumbar discectomy: clinical response in an initial cohort of fifty consective patients with chronic radicular pain. Pain Pract 2004;4(1): 19–29.

[36] Alo KM, Wright RE, Sutcliffe J, et al. Percutaneous lumbar discectomy: one-year follow-up in an intial cohort of fifty consective patients with chronic radicular pain. Pain Pract 2005;5(2): 116–24.

[37] Stevens CD, Dubois RW, Larequi-Lauber T. Efficacy of lumbar discectomy and percutaneous treatments for lumbar disc herniation. Soz Praventivmed 1997;42:367–79.

[38] Carey TS, Garrett J, Jackman A, et al. The outcomes and costs of care for acute low back pain among patients seen by primary care practitioners, chiropractors, and orthopedic surgeons. N Engl J Med 1995;333(14): 913–7.

[39] Frymoyer JW, Cats-Baril WL. An overview of the incidences and costs of low back pain. Orthop Clin North Am 1991;22(2):263–71.

[40] Takahashi K, Shima I, Porter RW. Nerve root pressure in lumbar disc herniation. Spine 1999; 24(19):2003–6.

[41] Carragee EJ, Han MY, Suen PW, et al. Clinical outcomes after lumbar discectomy for sciatica: the effects of fragment type and annular competence. J Bone Joint Surg Am;85(1):102–8.

[42] Waguespack A, Schofferman J, Slosar P, et al. Etiology of long-term failures of lumbar spine surgery. Pain Med 2002;3(1):18–22.

[43] Slipman CW, Shin CH, Patel RK, et al. Etiologies of failed back surgery syndrome. Pain Med 2002; 3(3):200–14.

[44] Rowlingson J. Epidural steroids in treating failed back surgery syndrome. Anesth Analg 1999; 88(2):240–2.

[45] Anderson VC, Israel Z. Failed back surgery syndrome. Curr Rev Pain 2000;4(2):105–11.

[46] Alò K, Wright R. First human dekompression: case report of 2-year follow-up. poster and oral presentation at the European Society of Regional Anesthesia meeting Spanish chapter, Oviedo (Spain); October 2, 2003.

[47] Kambin P, Brager MD. Percutaneous posterolateral discectomy. Anatomy and mechanism. Clin Orthop Relat Res 1987;223:145–54.

[48] Sasaki M, Takahashi T, Miyahara K, et al. Effects on chondroitinase ABC on intradiscal pressure in sheep: an in vivo study. Spine 2001;26(5):463–8.

[49] Hijikata S, Yamagishi M, Nakayama T, et al. Percutaneous discectomy: a new treatment for lumbar disc herniation. J Toden Hosp 1975;5:5–13.

[50] Onik G, Mooney V, Maroon JC, et al. Automated percutaneous discectomy: a prospective multi-instutional study. Neurosurgery 1990;26(2): 228–32.

[51] Javid MJ, Nordby EJ, Ford LT, et al. Safety and efficacy of chymopapain (Chymodiactin) in herniated nucleus pulposus with sciatica. Results of a randomized, double-blind study. JAMA 1983; 249(18):2489–94.

[52] Karasek M, Bogduk N. Twelve-month follow-up of a controlled trial of intradiscal thermal annuloplasty for back pain due to internal disc disruption. Spine 2000;25(20):2601–7.

[53] Bogduk N, Karasek M. Two-year follow-up of a controlled trial of intradiscal electrothermal annuloplasty for chronic low back pain resulting from internal disc disruption. Spine J 2002;2(5): 343–50.

[54] Nerubay J, Caspi I, Levinkopf M, et al. Percutaneous laser nucleolysis of the intervertebral lumbar disc. An experimental study. Clin Orthop Relat Res 1997;337:42–4.

[55] Degobbis A, Crucil M, Alberti M, et al. A long-term review of 50 patients out of 506 treated with automated percutaneous nucleotomy according to Onik for lumbar-sacral disc herniation. Acta Neurochir Suppl 2005;92:103–5.

[56] Bocchi L, Ferrata P, Passarello F. The Onik method of automated percutaneous lumbar diskectomy (A.P.L.D.). Criteria of selection, technique, and evaluation of results. Ital J Orthop Traumatol 1991;17(1):5–21.

[57] Alo K, Wright R, Fu ZJ. Open human torso laboratory dissection with annular and nuclear lumbar disc analysis pre and post Dekompressor®. Denver (CO): University of Colorado Health Sciences Center College of Medicine, Department of Anatomy; January 19–20, 2003.

[58] Wright R. Preclinical laboratory analysis of Dekompressor® percutaneous decompression in sheep and human cadaver discs: internal data. Fort Collins (CO): Colorado State University; May 2000.

[59] Manchikanti L, Pampati V, Fellows B, et al. Prevalence of lumbar facet joint pain in chronic low back pain. Pain Physician 1999;2(3): 59–64.

[60] Marks RC, Houston T, Thulborne T. Facet joint injection and facet nerve block: a randomised comparison in 86 patients with chronic low back pain. Pain 1992;49(3):325–8.

[61] Mooney V, Robertson J. The facet syndrome. Clin Orthop 1976;115:149–56.

[62] Suseki K, Takahashi Y, Takahashi K, et al. Innervation of the lumbar facet joints: origins and functions. Spine 1997;22(5):477–85.

[63] Bodguk N. International spinal injection society guidelines for the performance of spinal injection procedures. Part 1: zygapophysial joint blocks. Clin J Pain 1997;13(4):286–92.

[64] Kanpolat Y, Savas A, Bekar A, et al. Percutaneous controlled radiofrequency trigeminal rhizotomy for the treatment of idiopathic trigeminal neuralgia: 25-year experience with 1600 patients. Neurosurgery 2001;48(3): 524–34.

[65] Aprill C, Bogduk N, Dreyfuss P, et al. Percutaneous radiofrequency lumbar medial branch neurotomy. In: Bogduk N, editor. Practice guidelines: spinal diagnostics and treatment procedures. San Francisco (CA): International Spine Intervention Society; 2004. p. 188–218.

[66] Derby R, Lee CH. The efficacy of a two needle electrode technique in percutaneous radiofrequency rhizotomy: an investigational laboratory study in an animal model. Pain Physician 2006; 9(3):207–13.

**ELSEVIER
SAUNDERS**

MAGNETIC
RESONANCE
IMAGING CLINICS

Magn Reson Imaging Clin N Am 15 (2007) 273–276

Index

Note: Page numbers of article titles are in **boldface** type.

1064-9689/07/$ – see front matter © 2007 Elsevier Inc. All rights reserved.
mri.theclinics.com

doi:10.1016/S1064-9689(07)00068-2

Moving?

Make sure your subscription moves with you!

To notify us of your new address, find your **Clinics Account Number** (located on your mailing label above your name), and contact customer service at:

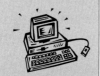

E-mail: elspcs@elsevier.com

800-654-2452 (subscribers in the U.S. & Canada)
407-345-4000 (subscribers outside of the U.S. & Canada)

Fax number: 407-363-9661

Elsevier Periodicals Customer Service
6277 Sea Harbor Drive
Orlando, FL 32887-4800

*To ensure uninterrupted delivery of your subscription, please notify us at least 4 weeks in advance of move.